D1606156

A Long Way from Home

McGill-Queen's/Hannah Institute Studies in the
History of Medicine, Health, and Society
Series Editors: S.O. Freedman and J.T.H. Connor

Volumes in this series have been supported by
the Hannah Institute for the History of Medicine.

A Long Way from Home

The Tuberculosis Epidemic among the Inuit

PAT SANDIFORD GRYGIER

McGill-Queen's University Press
Montreal & Kingston • London • Buffalo

© McGill-Queen's University Press 1994
ISBN 0-7735-1216-0

Legal deposit third quarter 1994
Bibliothèque nationale du Québec

Printed in Canada on acid-free paper

This book has been published with the help of grants
from the Canadian Federation for the Humanities,
using funds provided by the Social Sciences and
Humanities Research Council of Canada, and
Multiculturalism Canada.

Canadian Cataloguing in Publication Data

Grygier, Pat Sandiford, 1922–
    A long way from home: the tuberculosis epidemic
    among the Inuit
    (McGill-Queen's/Hannah Institute Studies in the
    history of medicine, health, and society; 2)
    Includes bibliographical references and index.
    ISBN 0-7735-1216-0
    1. Inuit – Canada – Health and hygiene – History.
    2. Tuberculosis – Canada – History. I. Title. II. Series.
    RC314.23.N6G79 1994   616.9'95'0089971   C94-900617-3

Typeset in Palatino 10/12
by Caractéra production graphique inc., Quebec City

This book is dedicated to my friend Margery Henson; to the beautiful lady in Clyde River who came to tell me her story, and to all those who suffered through the epidemic; and to the many workers who tried to help them through this difficult period.

Contents

Tables

Figures and Maps

Place Names

The names of most places in northern Quebec and a few in the Northwest Territories have been changed in recent years, and Inuktitut names have replaced those given by Europeans. I have used the present names of settlements except in direct quotations, where the modern name is given in brackets alongside the name used by the author quoted. The relevant names are as follows:

MODERN NAME	FORMERLY
Akulivik	Cape Smith
Arviat	Eskimo Point
Aupaluk	Hopes Advance Bay
Inukjuaq	Port Harrison
Iqaluit	Frobisher Bay, Ward Inlet
Ivujivik	Wolstenholme
Kangiqsualujjuaq	George River
Kangiqsujuaq	Wakeham Bay
Kangirsuk	Payne Bay
Kuujjuaq	Fort Chimo
Kuujjuarapik	Great Whale River
Quaqtaq	Cape Hopes Advance
Salluit	Sugluk
Sanikiluaq	Belcher Islands
Tasiujaq	Leaf Lake
Umiujaq	Richmond Gulf, near Little Whale River

Abbreviations

BCG	Bacille Calmette-Guérin (Calmette-Guérin bacillus) vaccine
CHUL	Centre hospitalier de l'Université Laval
DIAND	Department of Indian Affairs and Northern Development
D.Int.	Department of the Interior
DMR	Department of Mines and Resources
DND	Department of National Defence
DoT	Department of Transport
DPT	diphtheria, pertussin, and tetanus (inoculation)
DRD	Department of Resources and Development
EAP	Eastern Arctic Patrol
ENT	ear, nose, and throat
GNWT	Government of the Northwest Territories
H&W	Department of National Health and Welfare, Health and Welfare Canada
HBC	Hudson's Bay Company
IGA	International Grenfell Association
IHS	Indian Health Service
INH	isonicotinic hydrazide (anti-TB drug)
INHS	Indian and Northern Health Service
ITC	Inuit Tapirisat of Canada (national organization of the Inuit of Canada)
LIA	Labrador Inuit Association
MIVA	Missions Verkehrs Arbeitsgemeinschaft (a Roman Catholic international association begun in Germany to help RC missions in communication and transport)

MSSS	Ministère de la Santé et des Services sociaux, Government of Quebec
MSB	Medical Services Branch
NA	National Archives of Canada
NAB	Northern Administration branch
NA&L	Northern Administration and Lands branch
NANR	Department of Northern Affairs and National Resources
NHS	Northern Health Service
NWMP	North-West Mounted Police
NWT	Northwest Territories
PAS	para-amino-salicylic acid (anti-TB drug)
RCAF	Royal Canadian Air Force
RCAMC	Royal Canadian Army Medical Corps
RCMP	Royal Canadian Mounted Police
RG	Record Group
RNWMP	Royal North-West Mounted Police
TT	tuberculin tested (tested for evidence of past or present infection with TB)
USAF	United States Air Force

Acknowledgments

This book could not have been written without the help of a great many people, to whom I am very much indebted. First among these are the participants in the events, Inuit and others, who allowed me to interview them and who exposed their often painful memories to tell the story. Their names are listed in appendix 2, and I am most grateful to them for their time, understanding, and frankness. All the people approached for information were helpful, some for their stories, some for background information or contacts, and some for disabusing my misperceptions or giving a feeling for the flavour of a world I never experienced.

Secondly, I am grateful to the people who took part in the questionnaire study in the hamlets. Because of the nature of the study, the participants were anonymous, but I want to thank them, the students who interviewed them, and the staff who made the arrangements and supervised them from the following schools: Qitiqliq School, Arviat; Quqshuun Ilihakvik Centre, Gjoa Haven; the Gordon Robertson Education Centre, Iqaluit; and the adult education class, Arctic College, Resolute Bay. I am also grateful to the hamlet councils of Arviat, Coppermine, Gjoa Haven, Iqaluit, Pangnirtung, and Resolute Bay; to the boards of education of the Baffin, Kitikmeot, and Keewatin regions; and to the Science Institute of the Northwest Territories for allowing me to conduct the study in their jurisdictions. To all these people I am much indebted for the information they gave me. Most of the events they recounted took place thirty to forty years ago. Memory sometimes plays tricks, and what one person recalls may be at variance with what another will remember. I may not always have asked the right questions to clarify doubtful points, and I necessarily made a selection of the material available to me. Any errors in the retelling are mine, not the participants'.

My daughter Alexandra has been most closely involved with the writing of the book, and I am extremely grateful for her expertise. She started me on the archival research, herself doing the initial ten days' research on Record Group 85 at the National Archives of Canada. She then undertook a trip to the Northwest, collecting valuable information from participants and from various territorial government departments. She also checked most of my interview tape transcripts for accuracy and edited the final manuscript. Her help and encouragement throughout were invaluable. My son Jan initiated me into the mysteries of computers, advised me on the most suitable system, set up the program, and coached me through its intricacies. I doubt if I would have got very far without his help and encouragement, for which I am most grateful. Graham Rowley put me in touch with my first interviewees, opened his extensive library to me, corrected my initial errors in chapter 2 and, together with his wife Diana, has been a constant source of encouragement, practical help, and hospitality, for all of which I am most grateful.

The original impetus to write the book came from a talk by Brian Maracle on the CBC radio program "Open House." Subsequently, it appeared that this stemmed from an article in the *Calgary Herald* by Kirk LaPointe. To both of these journalists I am therefore indebted.

It is difficult to rank the contributions of the many others who helped, so I give them in alphabetical order. To all of the following I owe a debt of gratitude in one way or another: Alan Angmarlik, Pangnirtung; Dr A. Beauchesne, MSSS, Quebec; Anna Brancker, Statistics Canada, Ottawa; Patrick Burden, National Archives, Ottawa; Olive Gauthier, Archives Deschâtelets, Ottawa; Oxsanna Dzura, Cape Dorset; Martha Greig, Inuit Women's Association, Ottawa; Jack Hicks, Inuit Tapirisat of Canada, Ottawa; Robert Higgins, Inuit Tapirisat of Canada, Ottawa; Don Hilton, Department of Health, Yellowknife; Cpl Mel Hollett, RCMP, The Pas; Leah Idlout, Inuit Women's Association, Ottawa; Rhoda Innuksuk, Ottawa; Edna Lachance, CHUL, Quebec; Georges Lafleur, National Archives, Ottawa; Jocelyne Legault, National Archives, Ottawa; librarians at Hamilton Public Library, Hillfield School (Hamilton), London Public Library, St Marys Public Library, Stratford Public Library, the University of Western Ontario, McMaster University, and the National Archives, Ottawa; Winifred Lowndes, Lymm, U.K.; Dr Gillian Lynch, INHS, H&W, Ottawa; Dr R.A. Macbeth, Hannah Institute for the History of Medicine, Toronto; Jo MacQuarrie, GNWT, Yellowknife; Dr Roger McCullough, Medical Statistics, H&W, Ottawa; Dr J.F. McLellan, Agriculture Canada, Stratford; A. Les McDonald, The Lung Association, Ottawa; Winifred Marsh, Keswick; Sheila Meldrum, DIAND, Ottawa;

David and Suzanne Monteith, Iqaluit; Terry Newberry, Iqaluit; Barbara Novak, London; Chester Orzel, Hamilton; Dr W.A. Paddon, North West River; Lizzie Palituq, Clyde River; Dr D. Penman, H&W, Ottawa; Gary Pynn, Pangnirtung; John Rouble, NWT Teachers' Association, Yellowknife; Dr J.W. Scott, Grenfell Regional Health Services, St Anthony; Mrs Sissmore, the Arthur Turner Training School, Pangnirtung; Dr G.W. Thomas, Mabou; Dr F. Turcotte, CHUL, Quebec; and Doug Whyte, National Archives, Ottawa; and, finally, my excellent editor, Carlotta Lemieux, of London, Ont., and the staff at McGill-Queen's University Press, who worked so hard to bring the book into being.

If I have omitted the names of any people who helped in my research, I hope they will forgive the oversight; often I did not record the names of those who so generously assisted me, and I apologize for such omissions. Finally, I must apologize to the many people who could have added to the story had I contacted them. Time, energy, and money were all limited and, regretfully, I was not able to approach all those whose names I was given.

Introduction

In the 1950s the Inuit in Canada numbered some 10,000 to 11,000 people, strung across the shores of the Arctic sea and Hudson Bay or scattered among the Arctic Islands, up to 4,000 kilometres north of the big southern cities. They were for the most part seminomadic hunting groups, living in skin tents in the summer and igloos in winter, speaking neither English nor French but Inuktitut, writing in syllabics instead of our Roman alphabet, and having the most limited communication with the outside world – no telephones, no trains, roads, or regular air services, only limited radio, and a visiting supply ship and postal service once or twice a summer. Yet in 1956 the largest year-round Inuit community in Canada was situated in the Mountain Sanatorium in Hamilton, Ontario.[1] That year, the sanatorium was home to 332 Inuit patients,[2] some of the 1,578 Inuit who were being treated for tuberculosis in hospitals across Canada.

Tuberculosis had been brought into Inuit country by the European sailors and traders, and since the Inuit had no built-up resistance and virtually no medical services were available, the disease became of epidemic proportions by the middle of this century. After World War II, the Department of Health and Welfare mounted a concerted attack on the disease, organizing large-scale x-ray surveys and evacuating infected people to southern sanatoria, where they stayed for an average of two and a half years – though many stayed much longer. By 1956, one out of every seven Inuit was in a southern sanatorium. At least one-third of the Inuit population of the 1950s was infected with TB, and many required several lengthy stays in hospital. In some communities virtually everyone was infected at one time or another.

Many Inuit died in hospital and were buried in local cemeteries. Most recovered and returned north, though many were unable successfully to resume their previous way of life, either because of the physical effects of their disease or its treatment, or because of the difficulties of readjustment after so long a time in the south. Young children out for three or four years faced particular difficulties, for they had virtually become young southerners, who in many cases were unable to speak their parents' language and had no idea of how to behave in the demanding environment of a northern hunting community.

Since tuberculosis is a communicable disease, authorities can insist on an infected person receiving treatment. For southerners, facilities are many, communication is easy, family and friends are nearby for support, and language and lifestyle are familiar. For the Inuit patients, cut off from their northern communities, things were very different. Totally unfamiliar with a southern environment, usually with no money, and unable to speak the language, to communicate with the hospital staff, to contact their families left behind, or to return home without the authorities' help, the experience must have been as traumatic as it would be for a southern Canadian to be evacuated suddenly to a hospital in Russia, China, or Iran.

The effect on the families left behind was often devastating. For a people who were dependent on hunting in the Arctic, survival was largely a family affair. The men served a vital role as providers of food, and of skins for clothing and shelter. Without the women to prepare the skins for clothing and to care for the young children, the hunters could not function. And the children needed a long apprenticeship in the community to learn the survival skills necessary for them eventually to take over from their parents. Too much of any element taken from the family unit left all in jeopardy, and there was virtually no other employment – and no bank savings or unemployment insurance to help them through.

An immigrant myself, born and brought up in far warmer lands than Canada, I often wondered at the ingenuity and spirit that enabled a people to live in and enjoy the Far North; after only one Ottawa winter, I knew that I could never do so. After I retired and left Ottawa and moved farther south, I heard by chance a radio program about the Inuit TB epidemic, in which the broadcaster mentioned that no one seemed interested in fully recording the event. I was shocked by some of the patients' stories and was surprised that no comprehensive account had been written of this episode in Canadian history. Except for our aboriginal peoples, we are a society founded on immigration, and we need to relish every scrap of history we jointly have. So I decided to try to fill the gap while it was still possible to draw on the memories of the survivors. I was primarily interested in the human side of the epidemic, the effect the illness and the medical programs had upon the patients and their families; and I hoped that, in my analysis of the events, my experience as a clinical psychologist in Britain and the United States, and as a program evaluator in the public service here in Canada, might help to balance my lack of expertise as a historian and my lack of knowledge of the Inuit and the Arctic.

I was lucky to know a man who has many good contacts both in the Inuit community and among the government officials who worked with the Inuit through the 1950s and 1960s. Through him I obtained interviews with a few key figures in the programs, and they in turn supplied me with many more names as well as information. As the material from my interviews grew, I began to appreciate more of the difficulties faced by the government workers and doctors who had had to deal with the epidemic, and consequently I slightly reoriented my approach to the story and enlarged the scope of my research.

The research included a wide variety of sources: telephoned or taped personal interviews with former government administrators and welfare workers, with doctors and nurses, and with patients and their relatives; books and articles; the study of original documents from the National Archives of Canada; statistical tables and other material from Statistics Canada and the departments of health of the federal, Quebec, and territorial governments; a questionnaire survey in Inuktitut carried out by senior students in six of the hamlets; and a trip to the Baffin to visit some hamlets and meet some of the former patients or their relatives.

There was much material that I could not gather and there were many difficulties and frustrations: survey responses lost in the post; recording machines inadvertently turned off; the unwillingness of some participants to commit themselves or to reawaken old sorrows; the privacy regulations that required extensive work by the archivists before I could have access to the files; and the expense and difficulties of travelling, particularly in the Far North. Nevertheless, it seemed important that someone should gather what material could be acquired before the memories completely faded or the records were destroyed, and the majority of people I approached were most helpful and seemed appreciative of my intent.

This book, then, is an attempt to tell the story of the TB epidemic among the Inuit, to give a voice to the patients and their families, and to try to give a human face to the bare statistics. It also attempts to show the difficulties and effort of the many workers who tried their hardest to solve the countless problems they were faced with and who did, in the end, bring the disease under control and thus save the people from physical annihilation. This is their story too. The story is, of course, written with the incomplete knowledge of a southerner, who cannot hope to have a full understanding of this catastrophic episode from the Inuit point of view and who can only dimly perceive the impact that this massive event must have had on the communities scattered throughout the North and on the individual lives of the people directly affected.

All histories are incomplete, because the writer must select from the myriad pieces of information available – and in making the selection, one's own personal bias and the tenor of the times inevitably play some part, even if unconsciously. Another writer might make a different selection or have a different perspective on the same material. I have set out the facts as objectively as I can and have tried to identify the main threads running through the pattern of events. For the rest, the records and the participants will tell their own tale. It is, at least, a beginning. Perhaps an Inuk historian will go on to complete – or correct – the picture.

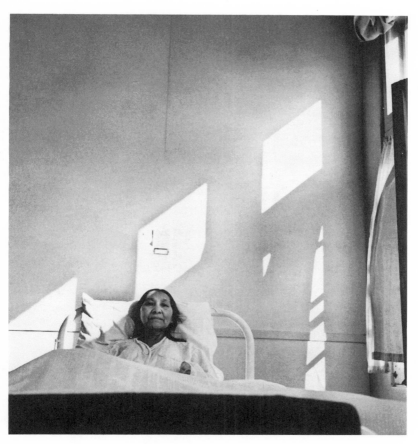

A patient at Charles Camsell Hospital, 1953. "Although she was small in stature, this Eskimo woman's serenity of spirit was not overwhelmed by the immensity of the hospital" (Yousuf Karsh, *Karsh: A Fifty-Year Retrospective*, University of Toronto Press, 1983, 0129441-F300-434 Comstock/Karsh).

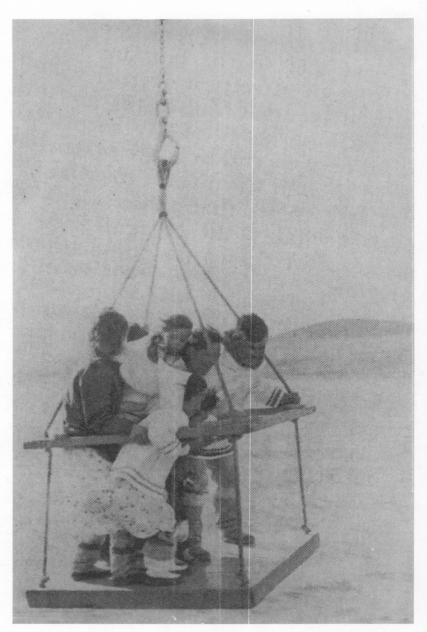

Another way of going aboard (G.M. Rousselière, *Eskimo*, Spring 1967).

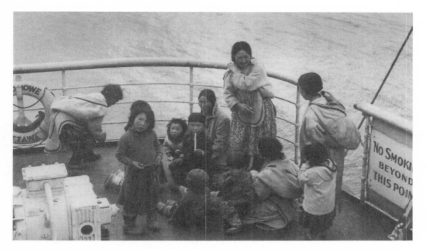

Aboard the *C.D. Howe* at Coral Harbour (W. Doucette/NFB/National Archives of Canada, PA-126552).

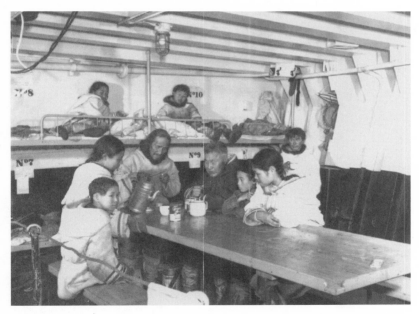

In the Inuit quarters aboard the ship (W. Doucette/NFB/National Archives of Canada, PA-176873).

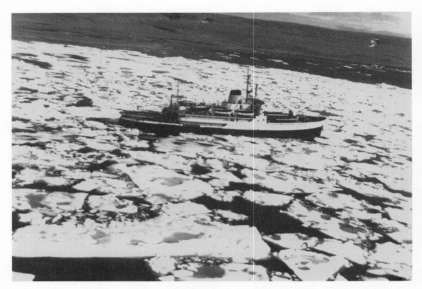

The *C.D. Howe* in ice at Resolute, 1959 (K.M. Parks/NFB/National Archives of Canada, PA-189644).

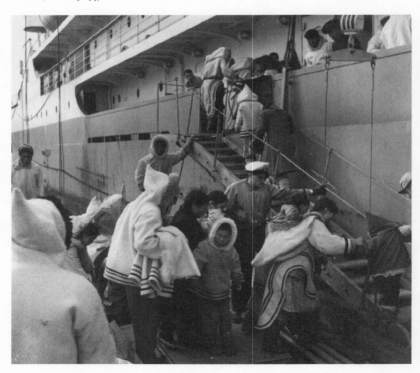

Boarding the ship in Lake Harbour, 1951 (W. Doucette/NFB/National Archives of Canada, PA-189646).

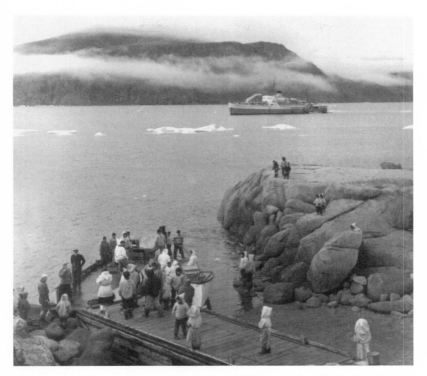

Arrival of the *C.D. Howe* at Pangnirtung, 1951 (W. Doucette/NFB/National Archives of Canada, PA-166472).

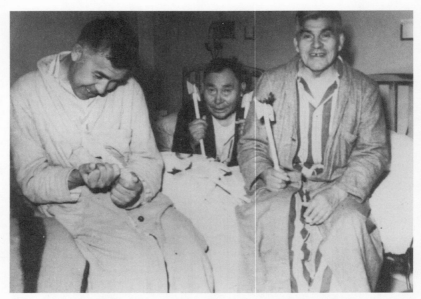

Men doing handicrafts at the Mountain San (Archives of Chedoke-McMaster Hospitals and the Faculty of Health Sciences, McMaster University. Hamilton Health Association Archive).

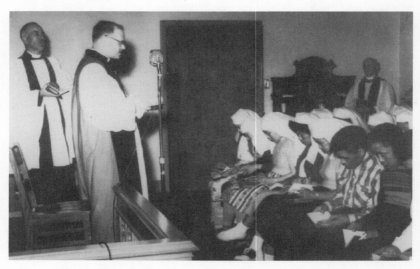

Bishop Marsh conducts a confirmation service in the Wilcox Chapel at the Mountain San (Archives of Chedoke-McMaster Hospitals and the Faculty of Health Sciences, McMaster University. Hamilton Health Association Archive).

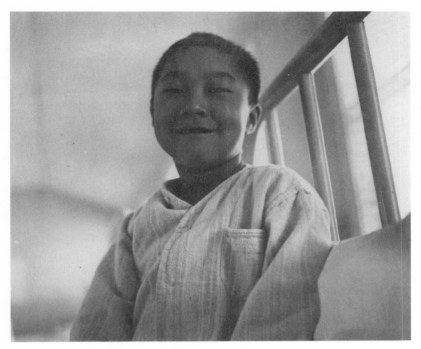

A young patient in Clearwater Sanatorium, Manitoba, 1956 (Gar Lunney/NFB/ National Archives of Canada, PA-189645).

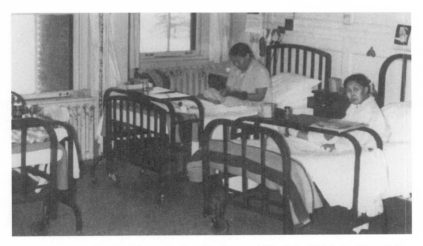

In a women's ward at the Mountain San (Archives of Chedoke-McMaster Hospitals and the Faculty of Health Sciences, McMaster University. Hamilton Health Association Archive).

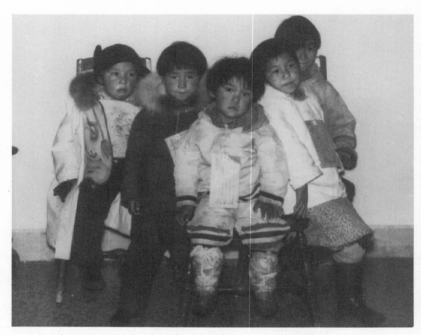

Five children just off the plane at Hamilton (Archives of Chedoke-McMaster Hospitals and the Faculty of Health Sciences, McMaster University. Hamilton Health Association Archive).

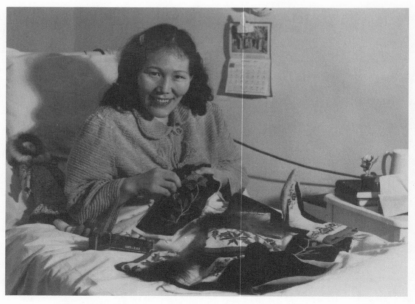

Annie doing handicrafts at the Charles Camsell (National Archives of Canada, PA-139314).

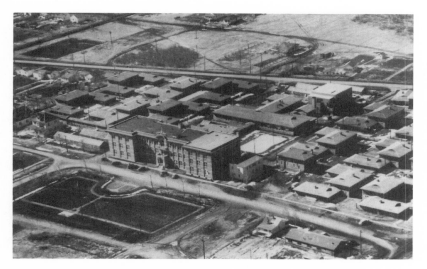

The Charles Camsell Indian Hospital, Edmonton, 1950 (National Archives of Canada, PA-139304).

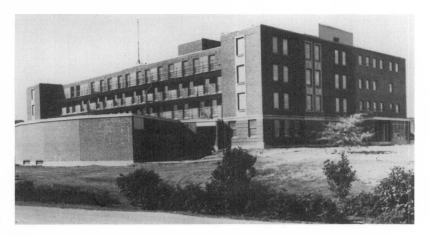

Wilcox Pavilion, Mountain Sanatorium, Hamilton, 1960 (Archives of Chedoke-McMaster Hospitals and the Faculty of Health Sciences, McMaster University. Hamilton Health Association Archive).

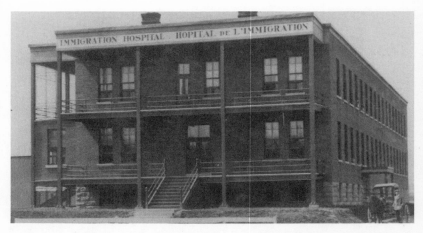

The Quebec Immigration Hospital, Parc Savard (John Woodruff/National Archives of Canada, PA-117288).

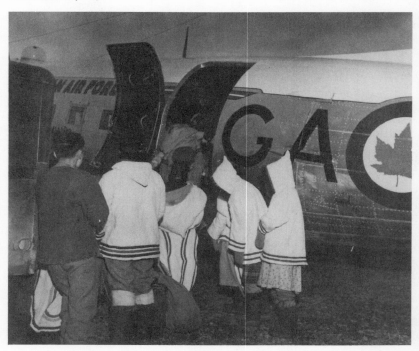

Sometimes they travelled by air (W. Doucette/NFB/National Archives of Canada, PA-189642).

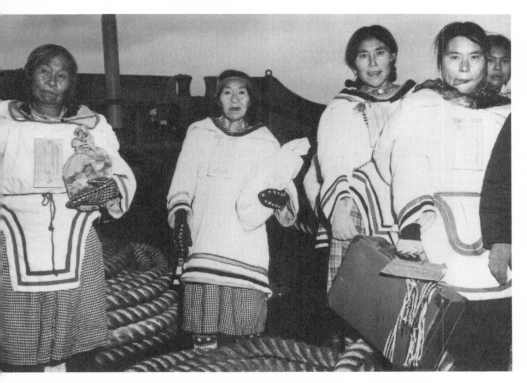

In transit (DIAND/*Inuktitut* 71, 1990).

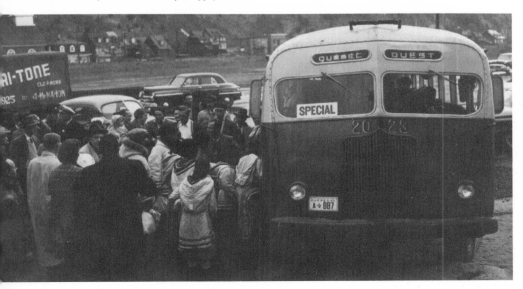

Transfer in Quebec City (DIAND/*Inuktitut* 71, 1990).

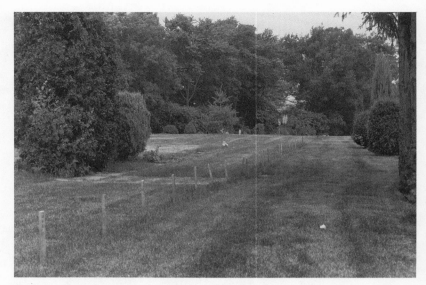

Inuit graves at Woodland Cemetery, Hamilton (Peter Bennett, *Inuktitut* 71, 1990).

Setting the Scene

A Brief History of
Tuberculosis in Canada

At the beginning of this century tuberculosis was the greatest killer of humans in the Western world.[1] In Canada it killed one out of every 1,000 people,[2] perhaps more, since not all cases were accurately diagnosed or reported. It was the disease for which there was no cure and was particularly prevalent in the slum areas and among the poor immigrant population of Canada's too rapidly developing cities. The attitude of the general public to the consumptives was much like the attitude of people to lepers in the past or to AIDS patients when this disease was first recognized – social disapproval, rejection, and, above all, fear of contamination.

As knowledge grew, attitudes gradually changed, facilities improved, and the death rate declined, but even as late as World War II tuberculosis was a major cause of death, particularly among young adults. Between 1939 and 1944 nearly as many Canadians died of TB (36,000) as died from enemy action (38,000), and the disease killed more people between the ages of 18 and 45 than all other infectious diseases combined.[3]

In the first 30 years of the century the decline in mortality was very slow, only down to 84 per 100,000 by 1926. But by the 1930s the many-pronged attack on the disease was beginning to take hold, and despite the effects of the Great Depression and World War II, the mortality rate dropped significantly. By 1950 it was down to 27 per 100,000. It then continued to decline until the mid-1980s, when it levelled off at around 0.5 per 100,000.[4] This decline partly reflects the much slower decline in the incidence of the disease, partly the introduction of mass x-ray surveys, which allowed the infection to be caught at an earlier – and therefore more treatable – stage, and partly the introduction of chemotherapy. But the TB death rate in Canada (around 8 per cent of those who catch the disease) is still said to be twice as high as it need be. Half of those who die do so because they were only diagnosed post mortem (and therefore never treated) despite, in the majority of cases, having been under hospital care for a considerable time before death.[5]

Accurate figures for trends in the prevalence of TB in Canada – that is to say, the actual number of people having the disease on any one day – are difficult to come by because the basis of notifications to Statistics Canada has varied over the years.[6] At first, figures were based on the reporting of new cases and on the number of patients in sanatoria and hospitals. Later, reactivated cases and patients treated outside sanatoria were included. The number of reactivated cases was about one-quarter the number of new cases in 1961 when the new system began, but this may not have been the case in the 1930s or 1940s. Tables 1 and 2 show the numbers of new cases reported, patients treated, and deaths, and the corresponding rates per 100,000 of the population, for the years 1938 to 1990.

Tuberculosis is an infectious disease caused by the bacillus mycobacterium tuberculosis and characterized by the formation of tubercles. The lesions occur mostly in the lungs (phthisis, or "consumption"), the intestinal tract, the lymphatic glands, the bones and joints, the skin (lupus), and the meninges of the brain (tuberculous meningitis). Tubercles as a rule proceed to abcess formation producing pus which, as the body's defences come into action, may slowly calcify and be surrounded by fibrous tissue. In this way the disease may be healed, and most older adults have the traces of childhood TB infections which their immune systems have managed to deal with.[7]

Sometimes the "cure" is incomplete, and the disease may become active again under conditions in which the person's defences are strained, such as another infection, pregnancy, or malnutrition. When many people are subject to situations resulting in a poor food supply, overcrowded living conditions, physical exhaustion – such as wartime, economic depression, or natural disasters – there may be many cases of reactivated TB and new infection of other people with lowered defences; in short, an epidemic.

Alternatively, the abcess may grow in size and eat its way farther into the surrounding tissues. If not halted, this can result in a secondary spread into other tissue through the blood stream or lymphatic channels. This septicaemia may cause a miliary, or generalized infection, setting up seedling tubercles throughout the body, a highly dangerous condition.

The specific infecting bacillus was first cultured and identified by a German bacteriologist, Robert Koch, in 1882, and it was then

Table 1
Tuberculosis Morbidity and Mortality, 1938–65

Year	Incidence: new active cases		Patients in hospital on 31 December		Mortality		
	Number	Rate per 100,000 pop.	Number	Rate per 100,000 pop.	No. of deaths	Rate per 100,000 pop.	% TB cases[1]
1938	8,936	80	8,661	78	6,172	55	69
1939	9,864	88	9,270	82	6,044	54	61
1940	9,804	86	9,772	86	5,845	51	60
1941	10,050	87	9,970	87	6,157	54	61
1942	11,532	99	9,943	85	6,061	52	53
1943	12,129	103	9,988	85	6,263	53	52
1944	14,702	123	10,244	86	5,853	49	40
1945	13,564	112	10,721	89	5,694	47	42
1946	14,307	117	11,771	96	5,941	48	42
1947	12,732	102	12,407	99	5,577	44	44
1948	11,561	90	12,950	101	4,887	38	42
1949	12,049	92	13,598	104	4,382	33	36
1950	11,562	84	14,930	109	3,679	27	32
1951	10,396	74	15,090	108	3,481	25	33
1952	9,537	66	16,047	111	2,538	18	27
1953	9,141	62	16,051	108	1,861	13	20
1954	9,122	60	15,220	100	1,593	10	17
1955	8,567	55	14,157	90	1,403	9	16
1956	7,930	49	13,072	81	1,256	8	16
1957	7,662	46	11,670	70	1,183	7	15
1958	7,215	42	10,425	61	1,027	6	14
1959	6,579	38	8,966	51	959	6	15
1960	6,345	35	7,755	43	823	5	13
1961	5,966	33	6,379	35	769	4	13
1962	6,284	34	5,189	31	785	4	11
1963	5,705	30	4,567	26	756	4	11
1964	4,541	24	4,085	23	670	4	12
1965	4,803	25	3,529	–	697	4	12

Source: Statistics Canada, tuberculosis statistics, morbidity and mortality, cats. 83–206 and 82-212, and health reports, cat. 82–003s10.
[1] Percentages calculated by author.

established that the reservoirs of infection were either human beings with tuberculosis or infected cattle. In 1890 Koch produced tuberculin by filtering dead bacilli, and although this proved to be ineffective as a cure, it is still used as the basis for a very accurate diagnostic test for tuberculous infection, the Mantoux test.

Human beings pass on the infection by breathing out droplet particles, either in direct contact or in coughing or sputum. Dried

Table 2
Tuberculosis Morbidity and Mortality, 1966–90 (Rates per 100,000 Population)

	Reported cases					Mortality		
	Incidence: new active cases				Patients			% of
			Reactivated	Total	under	No. of		total
Year	Number	Rate	(number)	(number)	treatment[1]	deaths	Rate	cases[2]
1966	4,497	22.5	768	5,265	10,796	669	3.3	13
1967	4,601	22.5	826	5,427	11,089	658	3.2	12
1968	4,824	23.3	755	5,579	12,498	630	3.0	11
1969	4,438	21.1	680	5,118	12,573	526	2.5	10
1970	3,920	18.4	620	4,540	10,716	527	2.5	12
1971	3,943	18.3	622	4,565	9,610	447	2.1	10
1972	3,908	17.9	571	4,479	9,019	453	2.1	10
1973	3,563	16.2	567	4,130	8,543	408	1.8	10
1974	3,354	15.0	416	3,770	7,380	330	1.5	9
1975	3,066	13.5	485	3,551	7,414	278	1.2	8
1976	2,722	11.8	421	3,143	7,371	264	1.1	8
1977	2,790	12.0	404	3,194	–	260	1.1	8
1978	2,549	10.8	391	2,940	–	220	0.9	7
1979	2,404	10.1	357	2,761	–	203	0.9	7
1980	2,446	10.2	316	2,762	–	188	0.8	7
1981	2,247	9.2	279	2,526	–	205	0.8	8
1982	2,200	8.9	273	2,473	–	196	0.8	8
1983	2,074	8.4	281	2,355	–	202	0.8	9
1984	2,091	8.4	265	2,356	–	182	0.7	8
1985	1,896	7.5	248	2,144	–	206	0.8	10
1986	1,900	7.5	245	2,145	–	182	0.7	8
1987	1,797	7.0	175	1,972	–	155	0.6	8
1988	1,771	6.8	176	1,947	–	160	0.6	8
1989	1,829	7.0	206	2,035	–	188	0.7	9
1990	1,787	6.7	179	1,995[3]	–	164	0.6	8

Source: Statistics Canada, tuberculosis statistics, morbidity and mortality, cats. 83–206 and 82–212, and health reports, cat. 82–003s10; Statistics Canada, Canadian Centre for Health Information, custom tabulation, 1993.

[1] Patients under treatment were not reported after 1976.

[2] Percentages calculated by author.

[3] Includes 29 cases of unknown status.

sputum may be a source of infected dust for as long as six months. The bacillus is not affected by freezing, but sunlight is lethal to it. People can get tuberculosis from infected cattle by eating the meat or drinking the milk. This used to be a major source of infection in babies and children, leading particularly to tuberculosis of the bones, glands, and intestinal tract, though any lesion is capable of spreading into other tissue through the bloodstream or lymphatic channels.

Once the sources of infection and the ways in which it was spread were known, an epidemiological attack could be made. In the case of bovine TB, the approach was to eradicate infected cattle and to use milk only from tuberculin-tested (TT) cows or pasteurized milk. To achieve this proved difficult, however, because of resistance from both farmers and public. The economic implications of testing all the cattle in Canada and then slaughtering those infected were enormous; and pasteurization was confused with boiling and thought to make milk less digestible for infants. So it was some time before either program was fully established.

Around the turn of the century, tuberculin testing was begun on breeding stock and on herds producing milk or meat for export. In 1905 a Supervised Herd Plan was introduced on a voluntary basis, offering free tuberculin testing of cattle but no compensation for any that had to be destroyed. In 1914 a municipal tuberculosis order was passed providing for the licensing of all milk vendors, the testing of cattle, and compensation for cattle slaughtered because of a positive reaction. In 1919 an Accredited Herd Plan was introduced, and in 1922 restricted area regulations were put into effect. These two measures in combination proved very efficient in eradicating bovine tuberculosis. To be fully accredited, a herd had to pass two or three semi-annual tests without a reactor. Under the restricted area regulations, all the cattle in a designated area were tested three or more times, with infected cattle being slaughtered after each test and the farmers compensated for the cattle destroyed. This provided clean areas for clean herds, into which outside cattle were not allowed unless they were negative on tuberculin tests.

In the early 1920s the number of tuberculous cattle found on the first testing of a herd in these circumstances was around 5 per cent. The second test produced around 0.5 per cent of reactors, and the third test 0.3 per cent or less. By 1954, some 80 per cent of Canadian cattle were in restricted areas, and in 1961 the first general test of all cattle in Canada was completed. By the 1970s, the infected rate was 0.1 per cent or less, and today the whole country is a restricted area with virtually no infected cattle. There are occasional outbreaks in isolated herds or in game farms, but with the continued testing program these are quickly brought under control.[8]

Pasteurization of milk, discovered by Louis Pasteur during his researches into beer diseases in the 1870s, kills the tubercle bacillus and, indeed, any pathogenic bacteria that may be present. A pasteurization plant was opened in Montreal in 1907, and pasteurization was required in Toronto in 1918. But pasteurization was not made compulsory until 1938 in Ontario and late in the 1940s in Quebec, and the pace was even slower in most of the other provinces. It has now been universally adopted. With the success of the TT cattle program and the pasteurization of milk, the transmission of bovine tuberculosis to humans in Canada has been virtually eliminated.

The attack on tuberculosis spread by humans was generally directed towards removal of the source of infection by means of earlier diagnosis and the isolation and treatment of infected people; by improving the social conditions that helped spread the disease and reactivate latent infections; and, eventually, by developing a vaccine to help prevent infections, and specific drugs against the tubercle bacillus.

In Canada the situation was at first made more difficult by the youthfulness of the country – the lack of organized public health services, the high level of almost unscreened immigration from the poor areas of Europe, and the still-emerging political structures (as usual, the federal and provincial governments were arguing about jurisdiction and responsibilities). But by the turn of the century, conditions were ripe for some progress. By then, the medical profession knew how the disease was transmitted and what circumstances most favoured a cure, though a cure could not be guaranteed. By that time, too, the public was thoroughly alarmed and was beginning to demand action of some sort, and the politicians had realized that the problem was a major one and was not going to go away without some effort. Most of the early progress, however, was due to the efforts of voluntary associations of doctors and concerned lay people.

In 1896 the National Sanitarium Association was formed, and in 1897 it opened the first sanatorium in Canada, the Muskoka Cottage Hospital. This was rapidly followed by various associations "for the Prevention of Consumption and other forms of Tuberculosis": the Toronto association in 1898, the Ontario association in 1900, and the Canadian association in 1901. The initial emphasis of these organizations (particularly the Canadian association, which became the Canadian Tuberculosis Association in 1923) was on the education of the public and politicians on TB, hygiene, and living conditions. The officers of the Canadian association lectured, wrote pamphlets, ran an anti-spitting campaign, urged the need for funds for sanatoria, and assisted in the setting up of local associations. The local associations in their turn pressed for more facilities than the general practitioners could provide, and from 1903 on regular tuberculosis outpatient clinics were set up in many general hospitals.

In 1895 a German physicist, Wilhelm Roentgen, had discovered x-rays which, as they were developed over the next 25 to 30 years, became invaluable in diagnosing internal diseases such as tuberculosis. Although the use of x-rays was hazardous with the early equipment, some Canadian hospitals soon started using them. Full dispensaries with laboratory facilities and x-ray machines were set up in Montreal in 1909 and in Toronto in 1914, and the first travelling clinic to serve areas outside major centres was organized in Ontario in 1923. As local health departments grew, they took over many of these clinics and added laboratory, nursing, and welfare services.

At first the clinics were limited to TB suspects and contacts, but gradually the wish to catch infected people earlier in the disease process led to x-ray surveys of people who were considered particularly vulnerable. Beginning in 1921, surveys were made of samples of schoolchildren across the country, university students, hard-rock miners in Ontario, and some Indian groups in the western provinces. Nurses in training, medical students, and teachers were among the early groups surveyed. Sanatorium nurses were particularly at risk; according to a Saskatchewan study, 60 per cent of female employees became infected with TB during their first year of service. In 1939 the federal government introduced x-ray examination of all recruits to the armed forces (and, in 1947, of people applying to be immigrants); one-third of 1 per cent of recruits were found to have active tuberculosis. In 1950 it became routine for general hospitals to x-ray all new admissions. Many previously unsuspected cases of tuberculosis were picked up in these surveys and routine examinations.

Meanwhile, treatment facilities also had been increasing, boosted by the need for beds for veterans returning home with tuberculosis after World War I. By 1925, Quebec and Ontario each had eight sanatoria, and there were one or two in each of the other provinces; as well, a number of general hospitals set aside wards for tubercular patients. Canada was a world leader in this aspect of the TB program, as it eventually was in controlling the disease. In 1953, the peak year for the country as a whole, the number of tuberculous patients in sanatoria and hospitals across the country was 17,364.

For most patients, the stay in hospital was long – six months to two years. The early sanatoria were usually built in the country, away from polluted air, visitors, and city distractions. Later, the sanatoria were located near larger medical centres and general hospitals. Bed rest, fresh air, and good nutrition were the main treatment in the first half of the century, but surgical interventions were also carried out – to remove tuberculous bone, for instance, or to collapse an infected lung in order to rest it.[9] From the late 1930s to the early 1950s, one in three patients with pulmonary tuberculosis had collapse treatment.[10]

Free treatment for all patients was first provided by Saskatchewan in 1929, followed by Alberta in 1936. Assistance programs were introduced in Ontario, Manitoba, British Columbia, and Quebec in the 1930s; and immediately after World War II, New Brunswick and Nova Scotia made treatment free. In 1948 the federal government started transfer payments to the provinces on condition that free treatment and the latest drugs were made available to all patients. Today, all provinces provide free – and obligatory – treatment.

The third prong of the attack on the human-transmitted disease was the development of an anti-TB vaccine. In the 1920s, Dr Albert Calmette and Camille Guérin of France developed the BCG (bacille Calmette-Guérin) vaccine, based on an attenuated virulent bovine tubercle bacillus. The vaccine was designed to be used as a way of raising the resistance of humans to TB when given before the disease had developed. There was some controversy about the use of a vaccine based on live bacilli, but it was eventually adopted, first in France and Scandinavia, and later in other countries.[11]

In Canada the vaccine was first tried on cattle in 1924. In 1926, under the auspices of the National Research Council, Dr J.A. Baudoin of Montreal gave BCG to 1,187 newborn infants from tuberculous families; he then compared their TB incidence over a 20-year period with a control group of 1,606 infants who did not have the vaccine, and he found that the death rate from TB in the vaccinated group was one-third that of the controls. In 1928 two doctors in the Indian Health Service[12] tried the vaccine on smaller groups of Indian infants in Fort Qu'Appelle, Saskatchewan, with even more striking results: the unvaccinated group developed TB five times more frequently than the vaccinated group; and among those of both groups who did develop TB, the death rate was five times higher in the unvaccinated group. Later, this vaccination experiment was extended to cover nurses and hospital attendants in Saskatchewan sanatoria, where there was a high rate of infection; and over a four-year period, the incidence of TB in the control (unvaccinated) group was four times that of the vaccinated group. However, such studies necessarily take some time to show results, and consequently the use of the vaccine was not general until after World War II.

The development of drugs that would cure the disease had begun as soon as Koch's identification of the bacillus had been accepted, but it was the mid-1940s before one was found. As mentioned earlier, the treatment of patients had previously been based on rest, fresh air, and good nutrition; it was very dependent on the devotion, flexibility, and persistence of the nurses, both in the sanatoria and in the public health field. In *The Miracle of the Empty Beds*, Dr G.J.

Wherrett describes the typical sanatoria routine which, as he says, was hard on both the patient and the nurse:

In the old days at Tranquille, BC, patients had to consume raw eggs and milk at every meal and between meals, and had to go out of doors in all kinds of weather, taking exercise under the close supervision of orderlies. This could mean a walk with bare feet in the snow. The routine called for a cold chest bath at 7 am, breakfast and dinner with windows thrown wide open, though the temperature outside might be 40 degrees below zero, and open-air exercise in the cold. At mealtime, a minimum of twenty minutes had to be devoted to the first two courses in a three-course meal.

There was a close affinity between long-term illness and poverty, and resources for help were few or non-existent. Consequently, nurses became involved in attempting to bridge the gap by soliciting help from voluntary agencies and groups to provide necessities such as food and clothing. Warm clothing was needed to outfit the patient for admission to the sanatorium, where he would spend the greater part of his time on an open porch to get the abundance of fresh air prescribed by the "cure." There was an added complication, too, since often by the time that the patient was ready for exercise, none of his clothing would fit because of the large gain in weight from the good meals and customary between-meal nourishment of eggnogs and milk.[13]

In 1944 Professor Selman Waksman and his colleagues in the United States developed streptomycin from a soil fungus, the first drug to kill the tubercle bacillus.[14] The effect was enormous. A disease that carried a mortality rate of 50 to 100 per cent suddenly became curable. Streptomycin was rapidly made available for clinical trials in Canada as well as in the United States, and its discovery stimulated the development of other drugs. At first the dosage levels were too high and caused serious toxic side effects, and the bacillus also showed a tendency to develop a resistance to the drug. But by 1950 appropriate dosage levels and applications had been worked out, and it was found that when streptomycin was used in combination with another antituberculous drug, the bacillus did not develop a resistance. Two effective supplementary drugs were found: para-amino-salicylic acid (PAS) in 1946, and isonicotinic hydrazide (INH) in 1952. Treatment with a combination of these three drugs over a period of 18 to 24 months proved very effective, and they are still widely used today.

Streptomycin has to be injected extramuscularly and is usually given in a hospital or clinic setting for about three months. INH and PAS can be taken by mouth and allow the patient to be discharged home at the end of the streptomycin course, so long as the pills are continued for 15 to 21 months. Other drugs have since been developed which give equally good results and are easier to take – for example, rifampicin and ethambutol – but they are usually much more expensive.

In Canada, until recently, an initial period of hospitalization was the norm for various reasons: to isolate the patients until they were noninfectious; to check for toxicity or drug resistance in the initial stages of the treatment; to build up the strength of the patients and to give them the nursing care they might need in the acute stage of their disease; and to coach the patients in the drug program they would have to follow after leaving hospital and in any adjustments to lifestyle that might help the cure or prevent a relapse. Today, only a minority of patients are admitted to hospital, most being treated throughout as out-patients. It is essential that the patients continue to take the drugs regularly for a year or more after they leave the hospital, and local clinic or public health supervision is usually enlisted during this period.

The rehabilitation of patients who survived tuberculosis used to be a big problem, at least for the ex-patients and their families, particularly before x-ray surveys allowed earlier diagnosis and treatment.[15] The treatment was long, draining an individual's or a family's resources. The disease (and sometimes the treatment, if it involved surgery) often left the patient with severe physical disabilities. Public fear often produced rejection, even of recovered and noninfectious patients, and there was always the tendency to relapse. Many people were unable to return to their previous occupations, particularly if these demanded physical labour; and social or emotional stress, economic hardship, or work that was physically too demanding led to many relapses. Even as late as 1950, one-quarter of the patients in the sanatoria were readmissions, and it was thought that half of these could have been avoided with proper rehabilitation. Continued invalidism and social support were the lot of many ex-patients.

As early diagnosis and therefore effective treatment became more frequent, more attention began to be paid to how the patients would fare in the future that had now opened up for them. Rehabilitation became a part of sanatorium treatment, and services were developed to help the patients. From about the mid-1940s on, there were available financial help, free treatment, in-sanatorium educational and vocational programs (instead of merely occupational therapy), and special post-sanatorium help through the rehabilitation agencies that were set up in all the provinces. In the more industrialized parts of the country, rehabilitation became easier because of the general shift away from manual labour to machine-assisted labour or white-collar work. In such areas as the Maritimes and the North, where the main employment is in arduous occupations such as fishing and hunting, the problem has been more acute. But even in these areas, it is now a relatively minor facet of the much greater problem of achieving economic diversity so that the general population can overcome permanent or seasonal high levels of unemployment.

Tuberculosis is a disease in which the emotional serenity of the patients, particularly if they are sick for a long time, is an important factor.[16] Two articles in the *Canadian Nurse* of 1948 dealing with rehabilitation programs for TB patients reflect the growing awareness of the importance of psychological factors in strengthening the patients' resistance to the disease. In the first, Dr Barclay McKone defines rehabilitation as "treatment of the patient until he may ultimately reach the maximum physical, mental, social, economic, and vocational capacity for future occupation and social security."[17] Dr McKone describes an experimental post-sanatorium program based on an appreciation of the effects of nonmedical factors on health and the need to treat the whole person instead of just his symptoms. The Veterans' Lodge employed doctors, nurses, rehabilitation workers, qualified teachers, occupational therapists, psychologists, social workers, and chaplains. A series of individual assessments of a patient in the first week culminated in a case conference, after which the patient was assigned to a course of his own choice. Adjustments in his program were made until the patient had identified the type of employment that would best suit him and had developed the skills necessary to work in that field.

Dr McKone also mentions the importance of planting the idea of recovery and rehabilitation in the minds of patients right from the start of their treatment when they first enter a sanatorium. This is the focus of the second article.[18] This is a reprint of a form letter given to patients entering the Queen Alexandra Sanatorium in London, Ontario, from the director of rehabilitation, Brenton Hellyar, who was himself an ex-patient, as were many of the sanatorium workers. While stressing health recovery and doctor's orders as the first priority for patients, the letter brings to their attention all the nonmedical services available to them and, by implication, their opportunities for future development. It describes the canteen goods and the bedside canteen-shoppers; chaplains and chapel services; patients' magazine, movies, radio programs, and earphones; the library with books, records, and visiting librarian; the education department with academic, vocational, and general-interest courses; the occupational therapy department for hobbies, such as needlework

Table 3
International Tuberculosis Death Rates for 1959
(Rates per 100,000 Population)

Australia	5.5
Austria	24.1
Belgium	17.0
Canada	5.5
Northwest Territories (mainly Indian and Inuit)	52.4
Inuit in 1962	73.0
Chile	54.6
Colombia	27.8
Costa Rica	14.5
Czechoslovakia	29.8
Denmark	4.0
Egypt	23.8
El Salvador	15.2
Finland	28.6
France	23.2
Germany, Federal Republic of	16.4
Greece	17.9
Guatemala	33.1
Hong Kong	76.2
Hungary	32.1
Ireland	18.2
Israel	6.1
Italy	18.2
Japan	35.5
Netherlands	3.6
New Zealand	
Excluding Maoris	4.5
Maoris	25.3
Norway	6.1
Panama	24.4
Poland	44.8
Portugal	51.1
Puerto Rico	29.2
Singapore	39.7
South Africa	
Whites	7.7
Asiatics	22.2
Coloureds	111.7
Spain	26.2
Sweden	7.2
Switzerland	15.8
Trinidad and Tobago	14.2
United Kingdom	
England and Wales	8.5
Scotland	11.1
Northern Ireland	10.2
United States	
Whites	5.5
Non-whites	14.4
Venezuela	23.8

Source: World Health Organization, annual epidemiological and vital statistics, 1959, from G.J. Wherrett, *Tuberculosis in Canada* (Ottawa: Royal Commission on Health Services, 1965).

and leathercraft; the exercise facilities and part-time jobs for convalescent patients; and the post-recovery rehabilitation and employment
services. Of course, the facilities varied from one sanatorium to
another, but the general trend to rehabilitation services was established and it may indeed have helped reduce the proportion of readmissions in the general population.

On the international stage also, programs of BCG vaccination,
x-rays, and drug therapy have considerably reduced the incidence
and death rate, though in most Third World countries tuberculosis
is still nearly as much of a problem as it was in the Western world
at the beginning of this century. The World Health Organization
reports TB as the second most prevalent disease in the world today,
with one-third of the world's population infected with it.[19] Table 3,
based on the annual epidemiological and vital statistics put out by
the World Health Organization, shows the death rates in 38 countries
at the end of the 1950s. It may be noted that in the countries with
multiracial populations where the statistics have been separated by
race (Canada, New Zealand, South Africa, and the United States),
the whites had markedly lower death rates than the non-whites.

There appears to be a link between TB and AIDS, and inadequate
supervision of long-term drug therapy in many poorer countries with
limited public health facilities has led to many patients stopping
taking the pills before the bacillus is completely dead. This, in turn,
has led to an increasing number of drug-resistant strains of the
bacillus which, with today's volume of international travel, can result
in outbreaks anywhere in the world, so that no society is safe from
the disease. And there still remain many centres of poverty in Canada
where such a seed once planted can rapidly increase.

So although the initial battle against tuberculosis has been won in
Canada, the disease has not been beaten, and indeed there are
increasing signs that complete control and eradication of it are elu-
sive.[20] The disease is on the back burner as far as general physicians
and the public are concerned, which may be one reason why some
cases are missed until too late. Given the right circumstances, it
could flare up – and sometimes does – and TB control programs,
education of medical staff, and research into new drugs and vaccines
are still important.

CHAPTER TWO

The Inuit People and the Arctic

The conditions in the Arctic before the advent of the whites into the society played a part in promoting an epidemic of TB among the Inuit. The intrusion of the whites, when it was solely for their own purposes without regard to the original inhabitants or the ecological systems of the land (for example, in whaling, trapping, mining, and defence), often not only introduced the infection into the population but also tipped the delicate balance of ecosystem and society, and brought disaster. When eventually help came, the characteristics of Inuit social and spiritual culture, so in harmony with the Arctic ecosystem but generally ignored by the Europeans, played a part in both the reactions of the Inuit to the behaviour of the government workers and in the psychological effects of the medical treatment imposed.

The Inuit have fascinated Europeans for a long time and have been written about – by foreigners – possibly more than any other race. But few people fully appreciate what it is like to live north of the Arctic Circle, let alone what it was like forty or fifty years ago. Although life in the Arctic is still hard and expensive, many of the facilities and comforts of the south are now available there. There are regular flights to most hamlets, albeit frequently grounded by storms. There is satellite television and prefab housing; there are schools and nursing clinics, postal, telephone, and banking services, fax machines, a largely wage economy, and many of the same goods available as down south. The territorial government operates much like any provincial government, with locally elected members (most of them natives) and a public service (mostly white). The Northwest Territories sends two members of Parliament to the House of Commons, and two Inuit[1] sit in the Senate. It was not like this forty years ago.

But first, a brief description of those aspects of the North which have not much changed: the people and the land. The Inuit are a specific group of people, or race, who share distinct physical characteristics, speak their own language, and have developed their own distinctive material and intellectual culture. They live in the Arctic Islands and along the northern coastline of Canada – including the shores of Hudson Bay north of Churchill in the west and Cape Jones in the east – along the coasts of Greenland and Alaska, and through the Aleutian Islands. The 1951 census of the Dominion Bureau of Statistics gave the Inuit population of Canada as 9,493, of whom 4,858 were in the Eastern Arctic, 1,999 in the Western Arctic, 1,789 in Quebec, and 847 in Labrador.[2] Comparative figures for Inuit outside Canada were: Alaska (1950), 19,774; Greenland (1951), 22,890; and the Soviet Arctic (1945), 1,300. It was a very young population: 66 per cent of Canadian Inuit were under 21 years of age (compared with 40 per cent for the whole of Canada), 33 per cent were under 11 years of age, and only 5 per cent were more than 55.

The Canadian Inuit all speak a specific language, generally referred to as Inuktitut, but there are sufficient differences between the dialects of the various regions to make it difficult sometimes for a person from one area to understand people from another. The Northwest Territories government recognizes six major dialects: Northern Quebec, Baffin, Keewatin, Arctic Coast, Western Arctic, and Delta.[3] In addition, in Canada the language is written in two different ways. Roman orthography, the alphabet used for European languages such as English, is used in the Western Arctic and Labrador; syllabics, an alphabet of symbols specially devised for native languages, is preferred in the east and around the shores of Hudson Bay.

In Canada, the Inuit occupy an area of about 2,500,000 square kilometres, so the population density in the 1950s was about one Inuk for every 250 square kilometres; or, perhaps more properly, since they mostly lived in small groups in crowded igloos, 20 or 30 Inuit for every 5,000 to 7,500 square kilometres, but concentrated along the coastal strip. About two-thirds of this land lies north of the Arctic Circle, where every year there is one day or more when the sun does not set, and conversely one day or more when it does not rise. Except for the Mackenzie Delta area, the land is above the tree line. There tends to be more snow in the Baffin and the east than in the Western Arctic. .

The coastal waters are open for only two or three months every summer because of the extremely cold temperatures. Some typical average Celsius temperatures for January are as follows: Cambridge Bay, high $-30°$, low $-37°$; Pond Inlet, high $-26°$, low $-35°$; Iqaluit,

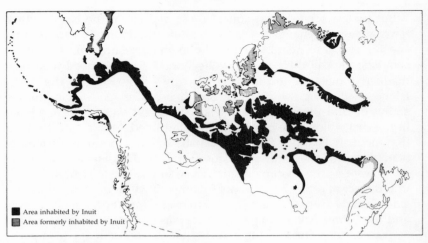

Map 1   Inuit Homelands
Source: G.W. Rowley, *What Are Eskimos?* (Ottawa: Information Canada, 1971)

high −22°, low −30°. Although the lowest recorded temperature in Canada was actually in the Yukon (−63°C in Snag on 3 February 1947), temperatures as low as −50°C are not uncommon in the Arctic. Except on rare occasions, even the summer temperatures are cool, despite the never-setting sun. July average Celsius temperatures for the same places are Cambridge Bay, high 12°, low 4°; Pond Inlet, high 8°, low 1°; Iqaluit, high 11°, low 4°.[4]

Winds tend to be strong, rising to 100 kilometres an hour during storms – a serious factor with such cold winter temperatures. Storms or fog come up with little or no warning, and there is little shelter so that in winter the winds cause drifting and whiteouts. Light planes can land on the ice or packed snow with skis in winter or on the water with floats in summer, but at spring break-up and fall freeze-up only permanent airfields can be used. In the 1950s the waters, like the land, were largely uncharted, and consequently sailing was particularly hazardous, even after the summer hydrographic surveys were accelerated. Navigation, for both ships and planes, was made even more difficult by the vagaries of the earth's magnetic elements in the Arctic, the weak horizontal component around the North Magnetic Pole (at present situated in the northern Arctic Islands), which makes a compass less responsive, and the especially violent magnetic storms, which produce irregular changes affecting compasses. Except within hamlets or in towns such as Iqaluit, there are even now virtually no roads; only in the Mackenzie Delta is there a continuation of the Dempster Highway, which links Arctic Red

River, Inuvik, Aklavik, and Tuktoyaktuk. All travel between other settlements must be by plane, boat, sled, or tracked vehicle of some kind.

Archaeological evidence suggests that Inuit or their predecessors have lived on their present lands for at least 5,000 years, having originally come from Asia across the Bering Strait. G.W. Rowley has described how the Inuit lived in the past:

The Eskimos had evolved a remarkable and distinctive culture that enabled them to survive under more extreme conditions than any other race. The typical form of the culture was the arctic form which was found among the majority of the Canadian Eskimos. Except in the summer it was an ice-hunting culture, based on hunting sea mammals either through the ice at their breathing holes, from the ice at the floe-edge, or on the ice when the seals lay enjoying the sunshine in the spring. The sea mammals provided the Eskimos with meat for food, oil for heat and light, and skins for many purposes. For this hunting the Eskimos had dogs and sledges and since there was little else to use in the way of building materials they lived in snow houses.

In the short summer, sea mammals were again hunted, but from kayaks and umiaks, or later often from canoes and whale boats, and the Eskimos lived in tents. At this time, too, fish were speared in the rivers and, more important, caribou were hunted, partly for their meat but particularly for their skins which provided splendid winter clothing. Nothing made in civilization is as warm, as light, or as comfortable for the Arctic winter as the Eskimo skin clothing.

This typical arctic form of Eskimo life was necessarily modified where conditions were not typically Arctic ... Though the great majority of the Eskimos lived by the sea, hunting sea mammals, there were ... areas where they developed an inland culture ... The Caribou Eskimos of the barrens [the western hinterland of Hudson Bay] lived almost completely on the caribou herds and fish of the interior, making fires from shrubs instead of blubber, and visited the sea rarely if at all.[5]

The first contact between the Inuit and Europeans probably occurred during the eleventh century, when the Vikings visited Labrador and possibly Baffin Island and fought with the local people. The next significant European contact was probably that of the British explorer, Martin Frobisher, who first entered the Canadian Arctic in 1576 and who met a number of Inuit on his three voyages. But as Rowley observes, "his relations with them were unhappy. He captured some of them, and they captured some of his men, and each side developed a hearty dislike for the other."[6]

Frobisher was followed by other explorers, who in turn were followed by whalers, fur traders, missionaries, and, in this century, by the RCMP, the mining companies, the military, and the federal government administrators. Each group of incomers brought new elements to the life of the Inuit, often affecting them adversely through depletion or disturbance of the animal resources on which they depended, sometimes offering greater ease or security of living through new technology such as guns or motors, and almost invariably introducing diseases that caused havoc in the communities.

To some extent the Inuit adapted to each new incursion – by crewing on the whaling boats, for instance, or trapping for the fur traders. Even so, they generally needed to continue hunting to supply their basic needs, and their customs and social life were not much affected by their periodic changes in occupation. Thus, as recently as fifty years ago, Inuit customs and social life remained much as they had been for centuries. The people lived in small groups of four or five families, sheltering in igloos or tents, depending on the season, and rarely settled in one place for more than a few months before going on the trail to hunt or trap the animals on which their survival depended. Each group had its preferred camping and hunting places and its overland routes between them, which were often marked by inukshuks – a particular arrangement of stones – to show the direction of the trail to the next sign. The groups usually returned to the same shore camp each winter, and travel was over the smoother sea ice as far as possible.

Despite the wide spaces and the scarcity of population, the people necessarily lived close to one another. The average family-sized igloo in an encampment (where a group might be living from about November until April or May) was from 4.5 to 6 metres in diameter and 2.5 to 3 metres high.[7] Large family igloos might have up to four cells, or smaller igloos, attached in line to the main one and joined by entrance holes. "Trail" igloos – which are still used by hunters today – are rarely more than 3 metres across. In the early 1950s, after the DEW-line stations had been set up, many of the Inuit homes near them were made from old packing cases insulated with snow blocks or simply snowed under. In some places, the winter dwellings were built of stone that was covered with moss and banked up with snow.

An igloo is partially dug out of the snow, and the entrance is low, so that one has to crawl down a small passage to enter it. Inside the dwelling there would be a low sleeping and sitting platform covered with furs; a small soapstone seal-oil lamp-cum-stove; a few dishes and cups, often enamel or tin, hanging from hooks or on snow shelves; a container for water, a large pot for making stew or porridge, and a frying pan for making bannock; and maybe a tin chamber pot. (There was, of course, no washroom – you went outside when you needed to.) An igloo demonstrates the inventiveness and survivability of the Inuit in their harsh environment. It was usually a snug and welcome place of safety in the bitter cold of midwinter. But, as Abraham Okpik put it,

This kind of shelter is fine and dandy but it is for a traveller who wants to have shelter maybe for one night or two when there is no other means of immediate shelter ... I am proud to be an Eskimo, but I think we can improve on the igloo as a permanent dwelling ... And when I say the Eskimo people need adequate shelter I don't mean the comfortable shelter some people believe the igloo to be, but a shelter like the rest of the Canadian citizens' houses ... The welfare needs of an Eskimo family ... are the same as anywhere else in the world, but more so in the north, because everything is so limited, especially in food, clothing and shelter.[8]

The changing of the seasons was always a particularly trying time for the Inuit. At the beginning of winter, the falling temperatures and great wet blizzards made the skin tents freezing cold and uncomfortable, and often ripped them apart or blew them away. But the snow was not yet sufficient or solidly enough packed for igloo building. Without just the right type of snow, the structure will not stand up to time and the rigours of the climate. Some groups built temporary sod houses to bridge the gap. Towards the end of May, when the igloos began to melt and drip, there was another period of discomfort; belongings and bedding would be damp and spoiling before there was sufficient dry level ground to pitch the tents.

Hunting, whether of caribou or seals, was an arduous and uncertain business. Seal meat used to be the staple diet of the Arctic Coast Inuit, and white fox and caribou the most important land animals, the fox for the sale value of its fur, the caribou for clothing as well as meat. The Eastern Arctic Inuit were more dependent on sea animals – the whale, the walrus, and the seal – but they also hunted caribou in the summer. There were devastating periods from time to time when the caribou failed to come or when the white fox, the staple "cash crop," was scarce because its main food, the lemmings, had declined; or when falling fur prices left the Inuit with insufficient credit to cover their needs at the Hudson's Bay Company store. Peter Freuchen, who lived for many years in the Arctic, described caribou hunting with the Inuit:

Hunting is not easy on the tundra – the endless, barren, flat land where there is no rock, no bush, nothing to hide behind. When the caribou stay together in herds they are safe because they have a clear view in all directions. To get at them one has to sneak up to them from a great distance, against the wind. After a while one has to crawl on the snow and finally to lie down flat on the stomach without moving and wait until the animals come close enough for the range of the weapons at hand. The caribou have very poor eyes, but an excellent nose. They get no clear pictures of fairly close objects as long as they are stationary. As long as the Eskimos don't move the animals may come within their range, but if they make one careless movement the caribou are gone ... In the days when they did their hunting with bow and arrow ... they might wait for days and days until the animal came close enough for the very limited range of their arrows, and they often had to return empty-handed ... Today the Eskimos all have rifles.[9]

The Inuit travelled because their survival depended upon it. Their existence was hazardous and insecure in the extreme. A lack of ice at the right time might mean starvation because fishing and hunting trips would have to be postponed. They had to be at the right spot just when they would find the animals that were most useful for their survival. They needed fat, which they could get only from the sea animals, which they also used for food, boats, and clothing. They found birds and eggs on the inshore islands. But they also had to go inland to fish in the lakes in summer and to hunt the caribou. The success of their trips was dependent on their accurate timing of the various animals' migration patterns. Disruption of these, whether by mining or military activity or by natural causes, could spell disaster for the group.

The very efficient material culture developed by the Inuit over the centuries to enable them to survive in their unforgiving environment was easy for the newcomers to appreciate. They had more difficulty in understanding the equally important intellectual and spiritual culture of the Inuit – and in many cases were probably totally unaware of its existence. Yet the full impact on the Inuit of the particular medical programs set up by the government to deal with the TB epidemic cannot be appreciated unless their social and spiritual systems are taken into account. The following summary is based on interviews with anthropologist Robert Williamson,[10] who lived among the Inuit as a student, as a welfare worker with the federal government, and then for twenty years as a professional anthropological researcher. Williamson has written extensively on the Inuit culture and its relationship to their language.

Traditionally, the Inuit have believed in the existence of a super-natural force or power, which envelops the whole of the created world. There is no belief in a godlike, humanoid figure. The power is seen more as a galvanizing and life-giving force, without which there is no life and on which all organic life depends – human beings, animals, and plants. The Inuktitut language uses the same word, "sila," for this force, for air (the most immediate necessity for life), and as the root for words denoting intelligence and thoughtfulness. This reflects the enormous importance placed on intelligence in their hierarchy of values. Intelligence, this creative force, is more important than physical prowess or material goods and is recognized wherever it manifests itself – in a hunter past his prime, in an old ailing woman, or in a young person full of vigour.

Also in the Inuit cosmology is the belief that each human being is the vehicle of a soul, which lives in that person for a time and is associated, indeed identified, with that person's name. The soul leaves the body when the person dies, but it may be recalled into another body by the process of naming. Hence, the naming of children is a highly significant event, and one's name has far greater meaning than mere identification. It is one's ongoing physical and metaphysical essence, one's personal reality. Similarly, if a person is sick, it may be that he or she needs a new soul, and hence a new name.

Souls are not linked to the sex of the person; each soul is worthy of respect in its own right, whether the body in which it is invested is female or male. So what comes out of the intellect of that person is worthy of respect as the product of a valued soul; and it is impor-tant for the group continually to renew the relationships with these valued souls in the kindred by reinvesting them, by naming them in newborn children or people who may be ill and need a new soul, or in admired outsiders who may be adopted into the group.

A characteristic feature of the traditional Inuit social organization, which at least partly stemmed from their particular geography and edge-of-survival life, was that they placed a much higher value not only on intelligence but also on cooperation and helpfulness than on self-assertion and competition. The communities were highly inter-dependent because, as Williamson pointed out, "no hunting camp could feel sure, however skilled or lucky in the hunt, *always* to bring back game. So even the best hunter was never assertive … People were not encouraged to be aggressive or assertive. Conflict between individuals could threaten the survival of the whole group." A cor-ollary of this was that women, during their child-bearing years, "could not draw attention to themselves and run the risk of becoming the objects of sexual interest and conflicts between men who were otherwise highly interdependent upon one another. Between their puberty and menopause they were very demure, very unforthcoming, apparently dominated by their male society."

Yet Williamson noted that the women were deferred to in decision-making situations at the family or extended-family level, particularly in situations where genealogical or kinship knowledge, or mythic, cosmological knowledge, was needed: "Women were the repository of a lot of this knowledge. And they were respected in direct degree to which they exerted their intelligence and judgment, and showed their characters." The old – men and women alike – were the repository of the family's wisdom: the treasure in Inuit society. According to Williamson, "they were the data bank, the source of knowledge and love. They were the bonding element in the society. Their ability to mediate between the physical and metaphysical world, between the natural and the supernatural, between the living society and the spiritual society, made them centrally important and beloved and needed." They gave the society both the sense of continuum and the sense of reality.

The Inuit's social organization and religious-spiritual philosophy seem to have been firmly based on their perception of the interdependence of all life, both within the family group and with their wider environment, and on the continuation of the group through the soul-name process and the knowledge resting in their elders. Of course, disruptions and disapproved behaviour occurred, as in all human societies, but on the whole their practical life and their spiritual, cosmological beliefs were remarkably well dove-tailed.

The literature and government reports[11] are full of examples of the difficulties of communication and travel in the late 1940s and the 1950s, despite the radio stations, Hudson's Bay Company posts, RCMP posts, and missions that were by then established at many of the spring and summer meeting places that are now the hamlets. For instance, Alex. Spalding, in his account of life with the HBC post at Repulse Bay in 1947, refers casually to the arrival in late March of an RCMP sergeant from Chesterfield Inlet, about 320 kilometres south, after a 16-day dogsled trip to bring the family allowance "cheques" (more accurately, store credits), which had just come in for the Inuit in Repulse Bay.[12]

Dr Otto Schaefer, who spent 1953–55 in Aklavik in the Western Arctic as medical officer to the two mission hospitals there and then spent 1955–57 at the mission hospital in Pangnirtung in the Eastern Arctic, described some of the problems facing doctors in the North:

Transportation is ... often a vital question for the few resident medical officers serving a native population scattered over vast areas of wild, trackless country. Two doctors, responsible for the Western Arctic Eskimos and the Indians and whites of the northern regions of the Mackenzie district and Yukon Territory, are resident in Aklavik; one in Chesterfield Inlet covers the northwest coast and hinterland of Hudson Bay, and one in Pangnirtung cares for Baffinland and Hudson Strait Eskimos ... The Indian and Northern Health Services have recently increased the number of nursing stations in the Arctic to ten. Besides these nurses, missionaries, R.C.M.P. and Hudson's Bay Co. personnel help most efficiently in emergencies as well as in carrying out public health programs and assisting in surveys.

At first I felt very frustrated on hearing emergency calls over the radio and often being unable to see the patients personally, for example during "break-up" and "freeze-up" periods, but soon learned to improvise according to conditions ... A memorable instance of medical teamwork took place in a small trading post on the Hudson Strait early in winter 1956–57, when a missionary, a Hudson's Bay Co. manager, a wise old Eskimo woman and a doctor, 500 miles distant at Pangnirtung, co-operated and removed manually the retained placenta from an almost fatally bleeding woman.

In the Western Arctic, we mostly used a small "Cessna" ... Needless to say, one had to adjust oneself to delays of days or even weeks due to bad weather, engine trouble or other hazards while travelling by aircraft, boat or dog-team. However, after my two-year term at Pangnirtung and approximately 3000 miles of dog-team travel over the rough sea-ice and tide-ice of the Baffin Island coasts and across wild mountain passes to the Davis Strait, even the old Aklavik of 1953 and 1954 seemed in contrast like a modern metropolis.[13]

Dr Schaefer also described some of the difficulties that the Inuit encountered when they sought medical assistance. In one incident, a man fractured his femur while fishing in mountain lakes, and his companions brought him in to the hospital at Pangnirtung. "Late freeze-up with much open sea-water and very little snow in the hills forced the party to travel a wide detour over indescribably rough, rocky terrain with the patient lashed for six days and nights to the sled in 20°F. below zero weather ... When I saw his badly displaced fragments, I wondered how he had survived his agonizing journey."[14] On another occasion, in June 1956, "a family arrived in Pangnirtung with an 18-month infant *in extremis* from meningitis after having travelled for a week from Hoare Bay across the snowfields, glaciers and, at that time of the year, the barren tundra and rocky gorges of Cumberland Peninsula and over the breaking ice of Kingnait fjord, where they had spent one anxious day and night on a drifting icefloe."[15]

Schaefer sometimes made emergency "house-calls," for instance in March 1956, when "a dog-team came racing into Pangnirtung from a camp 60 miles distant where a woman had suffered a severe haemorrhage," was unconscious, and was regarded as unfit for dog-sled transportation. Schaefer collected blood-grouping sera, transfusion bottles, and gynaecological instruments, and raced to the camp. There he grouped and cross-matched a number of people, transfused 1,000 cc of blood into the unconscious patient, and evacuated the uterus. As he explained, "All these procedures took place in a small, crowded sealskin winter tent, where the low ceiling kept my back bent all the time and the only sources of light were a dim seal-oil lamp and my flashlight. Next day we wrapped our patient in my sleeping bag and several caribou skins, and then transported her to Pangnirtung in order to receive more blood and antibiotics."[16]

In 1988, Schaefer said of his time in Pangnirtung: "I was perhaps the last physician in the Arctic who travelled by dog team, 2,000 miles a year. I can tell you, the difficulties were immense. The first year I was in Pangnirtung, which was the centre for the Eastern Arctic, we had the plane in three times, officially only one mail per year ... And I faced one epidemic after another that first winter. We cannot compare our times with then."[17]

Schaefer does not describe what it was like to travel by dogsled to do his emergency house calls, but it was certainly not a joyride. The lone nurses at the settlement nursing stations also had to visit outlying camps to treat patients, give immunization shots, and check on the public health needs of the people. The Indian Health Service director's newsletter of December 1954 includes a report from R. Horley, the nurse at Cape Dorset, on a January trip she made by dogsled with two Inuit guides, when she travelled some 320 kilometres across the Foxe Peninsula to Nunoodjuak, in order to check on two children believed to be sick with pneumonia, to inoculate the 60-odd camp dogs with rabies vaccine, and to check on the camp's welfare. The temperatures ranged from −40°C to −45°C, with a brisk north wind. It took Horley three and a half days to get there, half a day to examine the children and treat them with penicillin, to inoculate the dogs, and check the rest of the people in the camp, and then two and a half days to return to Cape Dorset. She and her two guides carried all their food and medical supplies with them and slept in trail igloos made by the guides each night. The report concludes, "Except for three frost bitten faces we had a very enjoyable and profitable trip."[18]

In her book *Lutiapik*, Betty Lee describes several trips that Dorothy Knight took when she was the nurse at Lake Harbour in 1957.[19]

Knight went primarily to immunize newborn babies and to give DPT follow-up shots, but she was prepared to deal with any other medical problems she found. Her medical supplies included five-day shots of penicillin, dental anaesthetic, aspirin, sulfonamides, ointments (including ophthalmic), cod-liver oil, vitamin supplements, and liquid DPT vaccines (carried in her inner parka to prevent them freezing). She also took standard first-aid equipment, some dental forceps, and a small enamel pot and strainer for sterilizing needles and instruments. Her personal baggage included a sleeping bag, prefrozen rounds of canned stew, pilot biscuits, butter, jam, a few cans of fruit, and milk, oatmeal, and tea. Her Inuit guide took chunks of raw caribou meat for himself and other meat for the dogs. Whenever they were to be more than a day on the trail, an Inuk woman accompanied them "for propriety's sake." They periodically checked each other's faces for signs of frostbite, for the temperatures were $-40°C$ (with the wind chill down to $-62°C$). For these trips, Knight wore a shirt, three sweaters, a pair of slacks, two pairs of socks (one heavy woollen, the other duffle cloth), high caribou-skin boots, a double set of mittens, and a caribou-skin suit consisting of pants, an inner parka, and an outer parka with fur-trimmed hood.

They travelled with the loaded komatik, or sled, on the snow-covered fjord, and at the beginning and end of each day's run they crossed the corrugated barrier ice between the land, where they built their night's shelter, and the fjord, where the going was smoother. Knight rode on the sled, sometimes getting off to jog alongside in order to keep from freezing. Once or twice a day they stopped for a mug of tea, a bite to eat (a slice of raw meat or pilot biscuits), and a cigarette. Each time, the dogs had to be unhitched and the sled unloaded and upturned while the primus stove boiled; sometimes the runners had to be re-iced and the sled then reloaded for the next part of the run. It was always a test of endurance for Knight: "Even through the sweaters and caribou-skins, she could feel the penetrating cold ... The trip was a nightmare of cold, boredom, and fatigue. When she stumbled beside the komatik, her body ached with weariness. When she sat on the sled, she gritted her teeth against the implacable cold."[20]

Knight and her Inuit companions usually set off at about seven in the morning, and they might make camp around nine or ten at night, depending on conditions and how easy it was to find snow suitable for igloo building. It was often midnight before the shelter was completed and they could unpack the sled, cook supper, and crawl into their sleeping bags; but at least they were warm in the trail igloos. By the end of two days, Knight "was only conscious of cold, exhaustion and the mesmeric hiss of runners in the snow."[21] On one windy trip they were in a whiteout and nearly lost their way, but were lucky to find an isolated camp where they were able to stay for a few days until the storm passed. On that trip they were away for about two weeks, and they returned to Lake Harbour without reaching the camp they had been aiming for, although they had visited three other camps.

Dr Schaefer suffered similar ordeals. He described the mixed blessing and sometimes devastating effects that military incursions into their territory had brought the Inuit. This was exemplified in the fate of K, a small camp of about forty people on the Davis Strait:

This group, living very far from the next trading post and blessed with a nearby walrus breeding ground, had subsisted almost entirely on native food until three years ago [1956] and enjoyed better health than most Eskimos living nearer to trading posts. Then a DEW-line site was constructed on the promontory above their permanent camp. The noise of dynamite blasting, planes and helicopters drove the walrus herd from their nearby breeding ground. The Eskimos could not move out, for all good hunting areas in our district were overpopulated. At first they enjoyed all the interesting new changes. Several of their best hunters worked for the whites and spent their money freely on cigarettes, radios and record players. They changed rather suddenly from an almost pure meat (partly eaten raw) diet to a predominantly carbohydrate diet. Their dogs starved the next winter for want of walrus meat. No travelling inland in search of caribou or hunting on the sea-ice for seals was possible with the few weak dogs left. Just that winter the build-up of the DEW-line site was nearing completion; all Eskimos in the camp were laid off and, in a belated attempt to save their dignity, all handouts were stopped at a time when they were really needed. An unbroken series of virus epidemics spread along the DEW-line early in 1957, and hit our camp K. particularly hard, consuming the last resistance in a population living in precarious balance with the ubiquitous tuberculosis. We evacuated on clinical grounds alone, in the spring of 1957, five patients from this camp, and the first roentgen survey in the summer of 1957 took another nine suspected cases of active tuberculosis south for hospitalization. Measles, after the shipping season in the fall of 1957, killed several more. By late 1957, almost half of the people living in the spring of 1957 in camp K. were dead or evacuated south.[22]

CHAPTER THREE

Other Players:

The Hudson's Bay Company and the Missionaries

The whalers arrived in the Far North in the nineteenth century and had a big impact on the Inuit. This was particularly the case with the American whalers, who stayed for two or three years at a time until their ships were full of oil and baleen. The Inuit crewed on their boats and learned a lot that was useful to them, but the whales and other animals on which the Inuit depended were overkilled and became very scarce. Moreover, the whalers brought tuberculosis and other diseases, against which the Inuit had developed no immunity, so the effect of their activities was generally negative.

The whaling industry declined at the beginning of this century and the whalers were gradually replaced by the fur traders, particularly from the Hudson's Bay Company, who spread north from their well-established posts in Indian territory. During the first part of this century, the three constant and long-standing influences from the outside world were the Hudson's Bay Company traders, the churches, and the police. In the 1940s and 1950s a typical Arctic year-round settlement consisted of a few Inuit families, a Hudson's Bay Company store (usually with two men), a mission (either Roman Catholic, with one or two priests, or Anglican, with a minister and his wife), and an RCMP post with one or two officers. The missions and trading posts were always established at places where there was a good harbour and where Inuit tended to come together because of a good supply of fresh food in the vicinity.

The Hudson's Bay Company (HBC) was incorporated in 1670 by Charles II of England and founded by his cousin, Prince Rupert of the Rhine, and other adventurers to trade with North American Indians.[1] The impulse was adventure and curiosity and the desire to beat the French in North American trade. This the company managed to do, and in 1713 the French were forced to acknowledge the

company's "title" to the region known as Rupert's Land. The acqui-
sition of North America by the British and their fight against
opposing contenders is another story, but in the process the Hudson's
Bay Company became a dominant force in trade and relations with
the original inhabitants of the northern part of the continent.

To carry on this trade, the HBC gradually set up a chain of trading
posts throughout what is now the Northwest Territories and regularly
sent boats into Hudson Bay, since this was the cheapest approach
from Europe to the fur forest.[2] As the boats sailed through the
Hudson Strait, they traded with Inuit of the area, who came out to
meet them in kayaks even as early as the seventeenth century. In the
nineteenth century, the company sometimes employed physicians as
its factors, paying them extra to treat diseased or disabled natives as
well as carrying on their trading functions. Although this practice
applied mainly in the Indian lands to the south of the Inuit, one
such physician was Dr John Rae who, during his time at Moose
Factory from 1848 to 1854, travelled widely in the Arctic around the
Hudson Bay and Keewatin areas and is said to have been the first
white man to live in the Inuit manner.

After Confederation, the Hudson's Bay Company ceded its territorial "rights" to Rupert's Land to the British crown, and these lands,
together with the area known as the North-Western Territory, were
transferred by Britain to Canada. Meanwhile, the company continued
its trading operations, though these had little effect on the Inuit.
Although the HBC had set up a post in Inuit territory, at Umiujaq,
in 1749, it did not have a permanent post among the Inuit until 1909,
when one was established at Ivujivik, on the northern tip of the
Ungava Peninsula. This marked the beginning of a major expansion
in Arctic trade. In 1912 the HBC opened a post at Chesterfield Inlet
on the west coast of Hudson Bay, and in 1915 it established the first
of three posts in the Western Arctic, in the Baillie Island–Mackenzie
River area. A year later, a post was established in Coronation Gulf.
This was followed in 1920 by a post on Ward Inlet at what is now
Iqaluit, and in 1921 by one at Pond Inlet in northern Baffin Island.
The year 1928 saw a new post at Coppermine; and so it went on.

Through the beginning of this century, the company tried various
schemes to garner the fruits of the Arctic through the work of the
Inuit. It organized a successful white whale fishery in Cumberland
Sound for a few years, but abandoned it about 1935 because of
depletion of the whale schools. In 1934 the company persuaded some
Inuit families to move from Cape Dorset to Dundas Harbour on
Devon Island to trap around there, but this failed because of the
severe ice conditions so far north, and most of the group eventually

ended up in 1947 at Spence Bay on the Boothia Peninsula. In 1939 the HBC tried to establish an eider-down industry on the islands off the south and east coasts of Baffin Island, but this also failed. Throughout, the company encouraged the partial conversion of the hunters to trappers, in order to fulfil the international demand for fur, particularly of the white fox. (The pelt of this animal is in peak condition in winter, and it is therefore trapped from November to May.) As a result, the Inuit's small winter communities on the shoreline, where they were accustomed to hunt for seal for winter food, were broken up as families stocked up with supplies from the company store and went off inland to their individual traplines for the winter. Even if the communities stayed together and the hunters visited the traplines on their own, there was insufficient time for hunting seals. So the people became dependent on the store goods – flour, tea, canned foods – which did not provide the vitamins, minerals, and fat which they needed and which their previous diet of raw seal meat had supplied. Their nutrition suffered, even in good years, and their resistance to disease was lowered.

With the new lifestyle and the introduction of the rifle, it seemed that an easier and more secure life would be possible for the people, but in fact they became rather more vulnerable. The rifle helped hasten the decline of the caribou in the mid-twentieth century, though the decline had probably already been set in motion by the military and mining activities. Secondly, the hunters' economic dependence on nature was merely transferred from one animal to another and was augmented by a dependence on the vagaries of world fur markets.[3] Thirdly, the people's unfamiliarity with the concept of saving goods or credits against a time of need – impossible in their previous conditions – and the absence of banks up north contributed to their tendency to spend their credits promptly, especially as they now had the opportunity to get things that were attractive, even though they had previously managed to do without them.

The company, of course, was in the North to do business and to make a profit, though in its heyday it seems to have shown a certain amount of corporate social responsibility towards the people it was exploiting. Many HBC employees became deeply committed both to the North and to its people, spending thirty to forty years in the Arctic and continually trying to improve the social conditions. Besides providing the supplies the Inuit needed (such as rifles and ammunition, food, clothing, and oil, which Inuit could obtain in exchange for furs or casual work for the company), the Hudson's Bay post was a source of advice and medical supplies; and after 1935, when the company began to equip all its northern posts with two-

way radios (before even the RCMP had them), it was also a source of
radio contact with the outside world. As well, from 1945 on, the HBC
posts were the channel for the store credits or food rations which,
for the Inuit, temporarily took the place of the family allowance
cheques for children that were being introduced in the rest of
Canada. In very difficult periods, when the animal population declined or the fur prices dropped, the company sometimes cancelled
debts or even gave its own welfare dole to the people. Since the
company was ubiquitous and the government representatives – the
RCMP – were very thin on the ground, the HBC managers often had
delegated to them government administrative duties, such as those
of registrar, tax collector, interpreter, and distributor of relief, thus
increasing their status in the little communities.[4]

That the HBC was often seen as a very negative influence over the
economy and life of the local population is shown by the reported
remark of one NWT administrator in 1931 that the only hope of
preventing the Inuit's eventual extinction was government control of
trading.[5] Happily, this prediction was inaccurate. Another view was
expressed in 1951 by Peter Freuchen, who stated that the Hudson's
Bay Company had done more than any other company in the world
to make life simpler and easier for people living in the North.[6]
Certainly, many of the managers worked very hard for the people
and were greatly loved and honoured by the Inuit.

Leo Manning was one such manager.[7] He joined the company in
Newfoundland in 1918 at the age of 15, and over the next 34 years
served with it all over the Arctic. He became one of the few whites
who were totally fluent in the Inuktitut dialects of both the Eastern
and Western Arctic. He worked at Cartwright, Labrador; at Lake
Harbour, Iqaluit, and Blacklead Island in the Baffin; at Inukjuak,
Povungnituk, Kangiqsujuaq, and Salluit in northern Quebec; and at
Aklavik, Bathurst Inlet, and Coppermine in the west. In 1952, Manning joined the Arctic Division of the Department of Resources and
Development as a translator and interpreter, particularly to help on
the summer Eastern Arctic Patrol. When it became known that he
was stationed in Ottawa, Inuit he had known when he was in the
company, or for whom he had interpreted while on the patrol, began
writing to him asking for news about their relatives who had been
taken south and not heard from again. It was partly due to Manning's
wintertime visits to hospitals to get the information to answer these
letters, and to his outcries in the department, that a Welfare Section
was started to try to deal with the social problems created by the
hospitalization program.

Missionaries have been operating in the Arctic even longer than the Hudson's Bay Company. The Anglican and Roman Catholic churches were the first to enter the Arctic, but the Moravians early established missions in Labrador, and more recently Pentecostal missionaries have set up establishments in some NWT hamlets. While the prime purpose of all missionaries is to convert people to their particular faith, those first working in the North found such a complete absence of academic and scientific medical services that these became a major part of their programs.

The Roman Catholic church is represented by the Oblates of Mary Immaculate, a religious order founded in France in 1816.[8] They first came to Canada in 1841 and spread through the Northwest, establishing missions among the Indians in what is now the Northwest Territories, the Yukon, and British Columbia. In 1859 they established a mission at Fort Good Hope on the Mackenzie River and from there made their first contact with western Inuit at Fort of Peel River in the Mackenzie Delta, where Father Grollier arranged a peace agreement between the Inuit and the Loucheux Indians.[9]

In 1860 the Oblates established a mission at a fur-trading post at Caribou Lake in what is now northern Manitoba, and from there in 1868 Father Gasté travelled northwest to Dubawnt Lake in the Barren Lands and persuaded the Inuit there to trade their furs at Caribou Lake. As in the west, this contact led to better relations between Inuit and the local Indian tribe, the Montagnais, and in 1906 Father Gasté went back into the Keewatin and spent seven months with Inuit of the Kazan River area. In 1910 Father Charlebois became the first vicar apostolic of Keewatin, based in The Pas, and in 1912, when the Hudson's Bay Company opened its new post in Chesterfield Inlet, he sent two priests north with their supply ship *Nascopie* to build the first Roman Catholic mission in the Arctic.

The Anglicans entered the Arctic at about the same time as the Roman Catholics.[10] They were early established at Fort McPherson at the edge of Indian/Inuit territory in the Mackenzie Delta, and in 1870 the Rev. William Carpenter Bompas went north from there to visit Arctic coast Inuit. In 1896 the Rev. Isaac Stringer established a mission at Herschel Island, which at that time was considered an unsafe place for a white man to live. It was one of the centres for the American whalers, whose impact seems to have been decidedly negative in the Western Arctic; indeed, their liquor law violations prompted the establishment at Herschel Island of the first Canadian police post in the Arctic in 1903. The missionaries were not always warmly welcomed. Bompas narrowly escaped death at the hands of

Western Arctic Inuit, and in 1914 two Roman Catholic missionaries, Fathers Rouvier and Leroux, were murdered by them.

In the east, Anglican missions were established at Churchill and Moose Factory, and gradually spread north from there. The first Anglican day school was opened as early as 1876 at Little Whale River by the Rev. Dr Edmund Peck, who wrote an Inuktitut grammar in 1883. In 1894 he established a mission and a second school at Blacklead Island on the Baffin and in 1895 a small hospital (which later closed) at the same place. Both denominations gradually expanded their missions through the Arctic. In the 1920s they rivalled each other by each building a hospital in the Western Arctic at Aklavik, the Roman Catholics in 1925, the Anglicans in 1926.

In 1931 the Roman Catholics set up a separate apostolic vicariate for Hudson Bay based on Churchill, with Father Turquetil, who had opened the Chesterfield Inlet mission, as bishop. By the time of World War II they had established a second hospital, at Chesterfield Inlet (1930), and missions throughout the Eastern Arctic – at Arviat, Southampton Island, Repulse Bay, Igloolik, Kangiqsujuaq, Baker Lake, Pond Inlet, Pelly Bay, Ivujivik, and Cape Dorset.

In the 1930s the new vicariate acquired its own supply ships, first a small boat called the *Thérèse*, which was replaced in 1933 by a schooner, the *Pius XI*. Then, in 1937, they had built a new steel 40-metre ship, again called the *Thérèse*, which was wrecked in the Hudson Strait in 1944. It was replaced in 1947 by the *Regina Polaris*, a converted minesweeper. The Oblates also began to use small airplanes, particularly for the inland missions, either those of the MIVA,[11] an international Catholic transport and communications organization, or those of the privately owned Canadian Airways; or, after the war, the Arctic Wings company.

In 1938 there were about 40 Oblates, most of them European-born, in the Far North. In 1952 there were 30 Oblates in a dozen missions and numerous out-stations in the Eastern Arctic alone, and there were still 29 of them in 1966. Their numbers have dwindled in recent years, as have the numbers of priests in other parts of Canada, and in 1988 there were fewer than 15 Oblates in the Arctic. But to a large extent they have replaced themselves by training lay Inuit catechists – married couples who teach the catechism, lead religious services, distribute the Eucharist, and are accredited by the government to register marriages. In the early days there were usually two priests, and sometimes a lay brother as well, at each mission.

As missionaries, the Oblates saw it as their first duty to preach the Gospel, convert the Inuit, and supply their religious needs. But they also seem to have equated conversion with the achievement of a higher cultural level, bringing peace and law to the people (who, ironically, had not even a word for war in their own language) by observing the laws of God. Even missionary activities primarily designed to help spread the faith often helped general cultural development. In 1917, for instance, Father Turquetil, who had learned Inuktitut in his time at Chesterfield Inlet, returned south to get a typewriter equipped with syllabics in order to print a prayer book, some hymns, and an elementary catechism in Inuktitut; and in 1919 he produced an Inuktitut grammar to help the Europeans in the North learn the language. In the late 1930s a Roman Catholic prayer book was printed in syllabics and distributed in the North, and in 1955 an Eskimo-English dictionary was published by the Oblates.

The two hospitals which the Oblates set up at Aklavik and Chesterfield were staffed by government-paid doctors and by the Order of the Grey Nuns, which was already well known in the Northwest Territories for its medical clinics and schools. By 1940, including the two hospitals in the Arctic, there were seven hospitals and two clinics that had been established by the Roman Catholic church in the territories.

In general, the Oblates seem to have supported the Hudson's Bay Company's fur trading with the Inuit, though they sometimes complained that the government and the company favoured the Anglican church. While often assuming the position of cultural and administrative as well as religious mentor to their flocks, they worked hard to fill the enormous gaps in social welfare in their communities. And along the way they carried on a vigorous rivalry with the Anglican missionaries and, later, with the Pentecostals.

In the early years, the Oblates survived by living as the Inuit did: hunting, travelling by dogsled, and seeing other Europeans (except the local HBC man or the RCMP) only once a year when the supply ship came in. The Rev. Hubert Mascaret of Chesterfield Inlet, who went to Ivujivik in northern Quebec from France in 1938, said of his early days: "It was a good life; we knew nothing else. I took it for what it was and learned from the Inuit about how to care for myself in the cold. While the Inuit were poor, we were sometimes even poorer. We lived alone in tents and snow houses. The Inuit had it much better. They had their women to tend to the seal and whale fat for their soapstone lamps."[12] Father Mascaret made his first trip home to France in 1950, and to do this he had to make a 30-day journey by dogsled, with 22 dogs, over the 1,600 kilometres to Kuujjuaq, where a military aircraft came in once every three months. He arrived with just six hours to spare.

Life for the Anglican missionaries was very similar to that of the Roman Catholics, except that many of them were married and were able to have their wives along for company and support, carrying out all the "duties" that ministers' wives everywhere usually take on. The Anglicans founded a mission in Aklavik in 1919 and built their hospital there in 1926, just a year after the Catholics, and in 1930 they too opened a hospital in the Eastern Arctic, at Pangnirtung. As with the Roman Catholic hospitals, the government paid the salaries of the two medical officers at the Anglican hospitals, and it also paid for a few nurses.[13]

In 1933 the Anglicans appointed Archibald Lang Fleming as their bishop of the Arctic. He had worked as a missionary in the North since 1909 and had been responsible for building the Pangnirtung hospital. Bishop Fleming saw a great need for hospitals in the Arctic and for many years pressed the government departments responsible to allow him to build other hospitals, for which he drew up plans and for which he had funds; but Pangnirtung was the only one allowed.[14] Fleming's successor, Bishop Donald Marsh, continued the struggle and later became a notable thorn in the flesh of the government administration.

The Anglicans set up schools as well as hospitals, both boarding schools, as at Aklavik in 1936, and day schools or part-time day schools in the settlements.[15] By 1937 there were seven schools. The Catholics had a boarding school at Aklavik and a day school and hostel at Chesterfield, beside their hospital; the Anglicans had a boarding school at Aklavik and day schools at Coppermine, Cambridge Bay, Baker Lake, and Arviat. Of course, these schools provided education for only a small proportion of the Inuit children, though some primary education was also given in other communities where there were missions, whenever the Inuit families gathered in the settlements; but no education was provided by the government until the late 1940s.

Apart from the bishops' attempts to establish hospitals up north, the Anglicans concentrated their main efforts on bringing the Christian faith to the people – as their confrères in the Roman church were doing – through the very practical process of teaching the syllabic system of writing and translating and distributing the scriptures. Between them, the two churches taught syllabics to such good effect that in 1955 Bishop Marsh could say that 80 per cent of Inuit could read and write their own language, a remarkably high figure considering the difficulties of communication and the paucity of schooling in the Arctic at that time (and compared with the present high level of illiteracy in "culturally advanced" southern Canada).

The Anglicans also put some effort into training local people to become religious leaders in their communities so that their Christianity should be indigenous. Their Cathedral of All Saints in Aklavik was consecrated in 1939, and by 1953 regular services were conducted in English, Loucheux, and Inuktitut.[16] The priest at that period was a Loucheux Indian, his assistant an Inuk, and the archdeacon a white man. After the Department of National Health and Welfare built a hospital at Iqaluit in 1964, the Diocese of the Arctic converted the hospital at Pangnirtung, which was no longer being used, into a training establishment for Inuit priests, who were ordained specially for work in the Arctic.

There seems to have been considerable competition between these two great Christian communions for the souls of the Inuit, and this may have spurred some competition in their provision of education and medical care. But they also saw it as their duty to work for the welfare of the people and usually found themselves, in the virtual absence of any other support substructure, taking on the roles of doctor, nurse, teacher, postman, social worker, and even radio-telephonist and meteorologist. They did this mainly for the benefit of the people in their local community, though they often did it for the government too. For instance, in 1927 the priest at Chesterfield Inlet built a radio transmitter, which proved invaluable for getting news, medical advice, shipping information, and so on; and the missionaries of Fort Good Hope kept daily climatological records from 1907 on.

The churches tried to fill the Inuit's needs as best they knew how and to the limit of their resources. If they sometimes overstepped their authority, some blame must attach to the lack of government concern and the vacuum that this left. A few priests of both persuasions seem sometimes to have become rather arbitrary and dogmatic in their assumption that they knew best what was good for the people. Many, being human, must have made mistakes. But on the whole they seem to have displayed the essential Christian idea of love of others – without judging, without asking anything in return, and without thinking of their own needs.

Both denominations set up industrial homes in connection with their hospitals, the Catholics at Chesterfield in 1938, the Anglicans at Pangnirtung soon after, and both Catholics and Anglicans in Aklavik by 1940. These homes sheltered aged and infirm Inuit, who would have been a burden on their seminomadic families and would have been at risk of death and in misery themselves on the move, especially at a time when the Inuit were finding it increasingly hard to find the means of survival. The government made more or less

Table 4
Diamond Jenness's Summary of "Medical Services, Schools, and Relief for Eskimo Territory for the Year 1939–40"

Item	Description		Cost
1	Medical Services. This item includes the salaries of four doctors and five nurses attached to the four hospitals at Pangnirtung, Chesterfield, and Aklavik; also their provisions, fuel, medical supplies, travelling expenses, etc.		29,480.00
2	Hospitalization of destitutes at the four hospitals		16,000.00
3	Maintenance of destitutes at the two mission residential schools in Aklavik.	20,000	
	Maintenance of destitutes in the Industrial Homes attached to the four hospitals.	6,000	
	Direct relief (provisions, etc.).	4,000	30,000.00
4	Grants to day schools at Baker Lake, Eskimo Point [Arviat], and Pangnirtung		500.00
5	Grants to the two residential schools at Aklavik, school books, freight, and express		1,750.00
6	Eastern Arctic Expedition. The main expense here was $25,000 paid to the Hudson's Bay Company for passenger and freight space on the *Nascopie*, as per contract		27,000.00
	Total		104,730.00
	Addendum: The Department paid for relief to approx. 1,800 Eskimos in Quebec Province		9,873.92
	Grand total		$114,603.92 [1]

Source: Diamond Jenness, *Eskimo Administration*, vol. 2, Canada (Montreal: Arctic Institute of North America, 1964), 70.

[1] Jenness noted that the costs at head office in Ottawa were not included in this sum.

token contributions to the homes, hospitals, and schools set up by the churches, but the cost of running them far outweighed the government subsidies. Some years later, anthropologist Diamond Jenness made a summary of the cost of medical services, schools, and relief for the Inuit, based on a statement which the deputy commissioner of the Northwest Territories had forwarded to the Indian Affairs branch in August 1939 (see table 4). In itemizing these details, Jenness commented:

I know of no reason why Item 6, "Eastern Arctic Expedition," should have been included in this statement, except that one of the four doctors listed under Item 1 joined the government party[17] on board the *Nascopie* to examine the health of such natives at the twenty-four ports of call as time and

Table 5
Diamond Jenness's Estimate of "Approximate Expenditures in 1939 on Eskimo
Education, Health, and Welfare, and on Police Posts in Eskimo Territory"

	Alaska (pop. 19,000)	Canada (pop. 7,000)	Greenland (pop. 18,000)
Education, health and welfare	$844,000	$88,000	$338,822
Police	$8,000	$119,000	–

Source: Diamond Jenness, Eskimo Administration, vol. 2, Canada (Montreal: Arctic Institute of North America, 1964), 71.

opportunity permitted. If we remove that item, the Department of the Interior spent, in 1939, $87,603 for the education, health, and welfare of some 7,000 Eskimos, which works out to slightly under $13 per head; and of that $13, health accounted for $7 (of which $5 went to pay the salaries of the field medical staff), education received $3, and straight relief used up the remaining $3.[18] Even the most casual inspection of these figures can leave no doubt that the administration was faithfully living up to its chosen watchword, "Economy."[19]

One might argue that this was in a period when Canada, like the rest of the Western world, was just coming out of the Great Depression and funds for social programs were necessarily scarce. But considerably more money was available for the suffering white population of the time. In 1934, for instance, the per capita cost for medical services for the white population was $31.

Jenness drew up a table comparing the amount that the Canadian government spent on services for the Inuit with the amounts that the U.S. and Danish governments spent on the same services, at the same period, for the natives of Alaska and Greenland (table 5).

Jenness commented: "What should we deduce from this table? Did the political philosophies of Denmark and the United States differ so greatly from Canada's philosophy that the first two countries could select doctors and school-teachers to be the apostles of western civilization, whereas Canada had to assign that role to the police? Or was Canada, as I believe, negligent? Did she choose the easiest path, the path of least expense, and give no thought to the reckoning that would come on the morrow?"[20]

Which brings us to the RCMP and the Canadian government.

CHAPTER FOUR

Other Players:

The Government and
the RCMP

The rights and wrongs of Canadian occupation of Inuit territory are not the subject of this book, nor is the government's general administration of the territory since it assumed control. But some appreciation of the Canadian government's policy and activities – or lack of them – in the Arctic is germane to its later handling of the TB epidemic.

After Rupert's Land and the North-Western Territory were acquired by Canada following Confederation, the Canadian government considered itself to be both the rightful and the de facto ruler of the northern lands. But apart from a few sporadic outbreaks of initiative, usually in response to a perceived threat to Canadian sovereignty, the government's behaviour towards the newly acquired territory and its native inhabitants might best be described as masterly inactivity. There was no military invasion of Arctic territory, no war was fought with the Inuit, and no treaties were signed; a few southerners simply arrived through the years, exploring or seeking the spoils of the country or propagating their religion. The Inuit continued in their accustomed seminomadic ways, living off the land, helping the strangers survive when necessary, and gradually making use of the new things they brought: rifles, groceries, a few medicines, a little teaching. But as we have seen, the Inuit were gradually drawn into trapping for furs or helping with the whaling in order to get store credits to exchange for the goods they had begun to relish and, eventually, to need.

At first there was room for all – and the Inuit way had always been to share the land and its riches. Although there were some murders and stealing of tools in the Western Arctic, the Inuit were generally tolerant and helpful towards the newcomers. As one pilot put it, they adopted the attitude "Here is another poor white man that we have to look after."[1] Perhaps only gradually did it dawn on them that the strangers had taken over Inuit land for their own purposes and considered it all theirs: crown lands – Canadian government property. But even had they wanted to, the Inuit communities were too small and isolated in their difficult climate to mount an effective opposition to the intruders.

The first action the government took in 1870 was to form the Department of the Interior (D.Int.) to take control of the new territories, which consisted of "all federal lands and natural resources on the Canadian prairies, in the Railway Belt of British Columbia, and the far North."[2] In 1873 the North-West Mounted Police (NWMP), the forerunner of the RCMP, was formed to police this area and assert Canadian sovereignty over it. Originally, the main function of the force was to control the developing prairie regions, to deal with the encroachments of American whisky traders, and to avert clashes between Indians and local settlers. Thereafter, the NWMP and its successors were the principal government representatives and agents in the territories; and as far as the Inuit were concerned, they remained so until after World War II.

The first twenty years of the NWMP were mainly devoted to maintaining order on the prairies and carrying out the policies of the government towards the Indians. But in the 1890s, with the growing mining activity in the Yukon, the focus shifted north, and in 1895 the first permanent federal administrative presence in the North was set up by the NWMP in the Yukon. More police and a contingent of soldiers were sent up after the Yukon was declared a separate territory, with its own commissioner and council, in 1898.

In 1903, in response to liquor law violations by American whalers, the NWMP established its first post in the Arctic at Herschel Island off the Mackenzie Delta, as well as a second post at Fullerton on Hudson Bay (moved to Churchill in 1906). Meanwhile, in 1904, the Mounties were granted the adjunct "Royal" and became the Royal North-West Mounted Police (RNWMP). In 1905 the Northwest Territories Amendment Act was passed, placing the districts of Mackenzie, Franklin, Keewatin, and Ungava under a commissioner and council, as had been done with the Yukon. But no council members were appointed, and the first commissioner of the new Northwest Territories was also the comptroller of the RNWMP, which continued to carry out the administrative functions in the field. Labrador, where some Inuit lived, was not included, because at the time it was a part of the Dominion of Newfoundland. The Canadian government had no jurisdiction over the people there until Newfoundland opted to join the Confederation in 1949.

The police not only enforced federal laws and regulations (especially regarding liquor and customs duties) and investigated crimes and captured criminals; they also

served as fishery overseers; licence and revenue collectors; mail carriers; assistants to Indian agents on treaty payment tours; protectors of Hudson's Bay and other companies' traders; wildlife wardens; customs collectors; mining recorders; coroners; justices of the peace; Crown lands and timber agents; forest fire wardens; construction crews (they blazed trails, wagon roads, and river routes); telegraph agents; and members of the two territories' councils. The NWMP officers on their extensive patrols also explored vast new stretches of the northern parts of the country.[3]

One government initiative in the period before World War I was stimulated by a disturbing report by W.F. King on *The Title of Canada to the Islands North of the Mainland of Canada* in 1905. The government responded by arranging the Northern Voyages led by Captain J.E. Bernier, 1906–11, and the Canadian Arctic Expedition under Vilhjalmur Stefansson, 1913–18. During this period, too, the Mounties set up a few more posts in the North and made several remarkable patrols, notably one across the northern barrens in the Keewatin in 1908, when they travelled by canoe from Great Slave Lake to Fullerton, thus linking the Mackenzie River system with Hudson Bay.

An even more notable patrol was carried out to investigate the reported murder of two explorers by Coronation Gulf Inuit. A patrol from Chesterfield Inlet spent 1914–16 preparing a trail and leaving caches of supplies through the northern barrens and along the Thelon River towards Bathurst Inlet. Then, in March 1917, an inspector, a sergeant, and three Inuit set off by dog team for Bathurst Inlet, where they arrived in May. They discovered that the explorers had themselves provoked the attack, so they made no arrests. Since the supply ship from Herschel Island, in which they had planned to sail on its return journey, failed to arrive, they had to return to the nearest police post at Baker Lake, travelling across the barrens by the overland route, which by then was mostly denuded of its caches of food. Carrying what supplies they could, they waited for freeze-up at Coppermine before they were able to travel further, hunting for food on the way.

The patrol left Coppermine in October but made slow progress because of the short daylight hours, the need to hunt, and a scarcity of caribou. By mid-December they were still in the barrens and were out of dog food. They abandoned one sled and killed five of the twenty-five dogs to feed the rest. A few days before Christmas they killed five more. Fortunately, just as they ran out of food for themselves, they saw musk ox and killed some, and then found one of the supply caches left two years before. Although temporarily relieved, they still had a long way to go and pressed on through blizzards. Food again ran low and they abandoned another sled and killed three more dogs and a litter of pups. By 21 January 1918 they had no food for humans or dogs. They cached everything but sleeping bags, ammunition, and rifles, and whipped the dogs on. Later that day they found caribou and shot ten of them. This was enough to carry them on to the Baker Lake detachment, where they arrived on 29 January 1918. They had covered 8,293 kilometres, all but 240 of them on foot, walking or running with the dogs, through practically unknown Arctic territory. Although this was the longest patrol undertaken by the RNWMP, they did many patrols of shorter duration and similar difficulty, together with their Inuit guides.

The concentration of administrative power remained firmly in the hands of Ottawa, with the deputy minister of the interior replacing the comptroller of the RNWMP in 1916 as commissioner of the Northwest Territories. In 1921 the discovery of petroleum in the Mackenzie district stirred him to fill the vacant places on his council. That year, too, the first local administrative offices of the federal government in the Northwest Territories were opened in Fort Smith.

The next year, 1922, the Department of the Interior centralized all the northern functions of the government in one unit: the Northwest Territories and Yukon branch. This consisted of two local offices, one at Fort Smith (for the Northwest Territories) and one at Dawson (for the Yukon), and four units in Ottawa, of which Eskimo Affairs was charged with the "provision of basic health care and the supervision of Medical Health Officers; education; sanitation; arts and crafts; support for mission schools and hospitals; and study of Inuit needs and habits."[4] To handle all this, Eskimo Affairs had between two and six staff members. All the fieldwork was still delegated to the Mounties (who had been renamed the Royal Canadian Mounted Police in 1920) or to Hudson's Bay Company factors or missionaries, or the occasional medical officer.

The Northern Voyages were reinstituted under the name Eastern Arctic Patrol (EAP) and were made one of the responsibilities of the Explorations Division. This patrol, which continued until 1969, gradually expanded and became one of the main channels for developing and administering the Eastern Arctic and one of the main tools for fighting the TB epidemic. But until the end of World War II, it was a relatively minor affair, consisting of a few federal government officials sent around the Ungava coast and the Hudson Bay and Baffin Island areas.

The first patrols sailed on the CGS *Arctic* or the *Beothic*, chartered from Newfoundland, but from 1932 to 1947 the patrol was accommodated on the Hudson's Bay Company supply ships, which visited their trading posts throughout the Eastern Arctic every summer. The duties of the government representatives were to report on the condition of the natives and the game, to adjudicate disputes, to carry out inspections, and to act as federal officers in various ways. The ship also carried a number of other passengers: RCMP officers and their wives, missionaries, radio or meteorological station operators and members of scientific expeditions travelling between various settlements, and usually a few Inuit who were moving between settlements or were going to or returning from hospital. A medical officer was sent on most of the two- to three-month trips to service the ship's crew and passengers and to give what help he could to sick people in the brief stops at the trading and police posts. The boat was primarily an HBC supply ship, with a tight schedule in difficult waters, and stops were usually for only a few hours, very rarely for more than a day. Little, of course, could be accomplished by one doctor in such circumstances.

Through the 1920s the RCMP set up more posts: at Pond Inlet in 1921, at Craig Harbour and Ellesmere Island in 1922, and at Bache Peninsula in northern Ellesmere in 1926 (later abandoned). In 1923 the first two judicial parties, each consisting of a judge, a crown counsel, and a defence counsel, were sent north to conduct trials, one to Herschel Island in the west, the other to Pond Inlet on the Baffin.

The year 1928 was a particularly busy one for the RCMP. An influenza epidemic hit the Herschel-Mackenzie area, affecting nearly all the local Inuit and killing 74 people. The Mounties, like the HBC factors and the missionaries, acted as doctors, nurses, soup-kitchen cooks, undertakers, and exterminators of starving dogs. During the winter of 1928–29 they took the census. During that year, too, the schooner *St Roch* was built and came into service in the Western Arctic as a patrol boat in the summer and a frozen-in base in the winter. Later, in 1940–42, this ship with her RCMP crew made the first west-to-east transit of the Northwest Passage, sailing from Vancouver to Halifax via the southern route. In 1944 she sailed the northern route back to Vancouver, the first ship ever to sail that route in one season. In 1950 she was sailed from Esquimault via the Panama Canal to Halifax, thus becoming the first ship to circumnavigate the North American continent. Her skipper, Sergeant Henry

Larsen, became the inspector in charge of "G" Division at Ottawa, and as such was responsible for all the detachments in the Eastern Arctic; he was later promoted to superintendent.

Through such activities, the number of RCMP posts was gradually extended through the Arctic, but by 1939 there were still only 28 officers across the Far North.[5] Fortunately, they found little need for their criminal investigative expertise among the Inuit, whom Larsen described in 1952 as so inherently honest that theft was almost unknown.[6] To help them, they trained and employed a few special constables from among the people. "G" Division, which covers the whole North, today has about 240 officers in 4 subdivisions and 39 detachments, most of which are headed by a sergeant or a corporal.

The police officers were on occasion called on to help in medical emergencies, sometimes following instructions from a doctor over the radio, and to transport sick or injured people out to places where they could get professional help. The Department of Transport was developing a system of radio and weather stations in the Arctic, and by 1937 it had stations at Coppermine and Iqaluit, in Hudson Strait, and on each shore of Hudson Bay; all were linked to telegraph stations such as the one at Churchill. By 1939, the RCMP had a single-engine Norseman aircraft based in the Mackenzie Delta to service the western detachments with freight and food, and to transfer members between detachments. During the 1940s the Mounties used this plane to respond to urgent calls for patient transfer when life-saving time was a factor. The plane also helped speed up criminal investigations. But usually, like the missionaries and the HBC managers, the Mounties used dog teams to make their patrols, and in the east they relied mainly on the HBC or mission ships to supply their posts.

Sometimes, informal and arbitrary justice was meted out by the police. Dr J. Moody, who was the doctor at the mission hospital in Chesterfield in the late 1940s, has described how an Inuk was brought to the settlement because the RCMP were suspicious about the death of his wife. Although an autopsy showed nothing definite, the man was not allowed to leave: the police decided to "keep an eye on him" in Chesterfield.[7] Moody observed that the Inuit often found it difficult to understand the southern laws and morals, which had evolved in a society in which their own problems were not known, their needs not felt, and their morals not understood. In today's Western civilization there is generally speaking no need, for instance, for infanticide or assisted suicide, but in Inuit culture these things had long been considered natural and were accepted as necessary on occasion,

though not performed without grief. The Inuit were therefore confused when charged with murder for such killings.[8]

The RCMP not only had to enforce the southern laws; they were, in
effect, colonial administrators in much the same way that British colonial service officers were in India and Africa. To this extent, Jenness's
table of the money spent on police versus education, health, and
welfare in Alaska, Greenland, and Canada (table 5) is a little mis-
leading, because some part of the RCMP time and money were spent
on health and welfare, at least in the period before World War II.

The Department of the Interior, meanwhile, under pressure from
the churches, had in 1922 appointed the first resident physician to
the Inuit, Dr Leslie Livingstone. He was an unusual choice for a
government doctor, but perhaps a good one for the Arctic.[9] He had
originally trained as a mining engineer, geologist, and prospector,
and although he completed his medical courses at Queen's University,
he never sat his final exam. It was only much later that the university
granted him an honorary doctorate in medicine. However, he was
largely instrumental in establishing the first government medical
service in the Far North.

Livingstone sailed on the Eastern Arctic Patrol from 1922 to 1926,
pressing in the meantime for the establishment of a land-based
service of the type that is now in operation; namely, small nursing
stations in each of the major settlements, offering out-patient services
and having a few beds, facilities for minor surgery, and a visiting
doctor. Livingstone moved to Pangnirtung in 1927 and opened the
first of his "medical headquarters" there in 1928, allying it with the
hospital that was being built by the Anglicans. That year, too, he
was appointed senior medical officer in the fledgling Northern Health
Service. By 1930, he had six medical officers under him and had
opened a second medical station at Chesterfield in cooperation with
the Roman Catholic hospital there. That year, doctors were in Inuit
country at Chesterfield, Coppermine, Pangnirtung, Aklavik, and (on
the borderline but serving the Inuit) Moose Factory.

As reflected in table 4 (in chapter 3), the Department of the Interior
agreed to pay the missions something towards the cost of hospital
care and schools for the Inuit. Under the Northwest Territories Act,
for instance, section 2 of the Hospitals Amendment Ordinance of
June 1933 provides that certain "hospitals in the Territories ... shall
receive such public aid as the Commissioner may from time to time
fix and determine."[10] Aid to the hospitals was given in the form of:

• grants towards construction of about 40 per cent of initial cost;
• equipment (discontinued by 1943);

- per diem allowance for indigent patients (since the Inuit society had a basically nonmonetary economy at that time, this applied to all Inuit);
- guaranteed minimum revenues (for Chesterfield and Pangnirtung);
- allowance for patients in industrial homes operated by the hospitals;
- transportation of building materials and annual freight;
- drugs and medicines; and
- services of a limited number of doctors and registered nurses (usually one doctor and one or two nurses per hospital). In 1935, for instance, the department paid for three doctors and four nurses at the hospitals in Aklavik, Chesterfield, and Pangnirtung, and the per diem allowance was raised that year from $1.50 to $2.50 per patient.

Before World War II, a doctor paid by the Northwest Territories administration was stationed at each of the following locations: Aklavik (serving two hospitals, the Mackenzie Delta, and most of the Western Arctic), Pangnirtung (serving one hospital and the surrounding Baffin), and Chesterfield Inlet (serving one hospital and the surrounding Keewatin) generally from the late 1920s; at Coppermine for a brief period, 1929–31; and at Moose Factory, which was primarily an Indian settlement but received some Inuit patients from the Ungava and James Bay areas, from 1930 on.

In 1931 the Northwest Territories and Yukon branch was abolished and its functions came under the new Dominion Lands Board, which also was in the Department of the Interior; and in 1934 the name of the Dominion Lands Board was changed to Lands, Northwest Territories and Yukon branch. But on each occasion there was no real change in the operations. However, in 1936 a major reorganization took place when the Department of the Interior was dissolved and its functions, including responsibility for Inuit affairs, were placed in the new omnibus Department of Mines and Resources (DMR), which itself was formed from a merger of three departments: Mines, Indian Affairs, and Immigration and Colonization. Inuit affairs continued to be the responsibility of a Bureau of Northwest Territories and Yukon Affairs (specifically, the Eastern Arctic Division of this bureau), but it was now under the Lands, Parks, and Forests branch of the new department.[11]

At the same time that Dr Livingstone was developing his Northern Health Service at the Department of the Interior, the Department of Indian Affairs was developing a parallel Indian Health Service under

Dr E.L. Stone, who had been appointed in 1927. When the responsibility for both Indian and Inuit affairs was transferred to the new department, the two medical groups were combined into the Indian Health Services (including Eskimos) division under Dr Stone. Dr Livingstone, who had for a long time been rather put out by D.Int.'s tendency to refer medical matters over his head to the doctors at the Department of Pensions and National Health, continued to work at Aklavik for some years as the district administrator, trying in various ways to improve the lot of the local people and hospital patients, for instance, by establishing a dairy herd and by stimulating geological surveys.

Under the Eastern Arctic Division fell the general administration of the Northwest Territories, the Eastern Arctic Patrol, and the provision of northern medical services. The division had field offices at Fort Smith, Port Radium, and Yellowknife. Where they were in place, the field officers at last gave the RCMP some relief from administrative duties: the field officer at Fort Smith was also the superintendent of Wood Buffalo National Park, dominion lands agent, crown timber agent, mining recorder, stipendiary magistrate, and marriage commissioner. The medical officers also were often required to do general administration for the department. For instance, the MO at Aklavik, besides servicing two hospitals, was the department's agent for the Lower Mackenzie and Western Arctic, and supervisor of the Mackenzie Delta reindeer industry.

The first hint of independence from Ottawa for the North came in 1939 when the Yellowknife Administrative District, under a partially elected Local Trustee Board, was established, bringing the beginning of municipal government to the territories – though many years were to pass before it came to the Arctic. Apart from the gradual spread of the RCMP posts and patrols, the main government activities that impinged on the Inuit before World War II were the annual Eastern Arctic Patrol and the limited financial support given to the hospitals and schools set up by the missions.

The situation changed radically in the 1940s. For one thing, Canada and Newfoundland allowed the United States to enter the area to construct airfields and hospitals at several points in Inuit territory or close by (Kuujjuaq, Iqaluit, Churchill, Goose Bay, and Southampton Island) for its northwest staging route, or Crimson Line. This established for the first time a military presence in the Far North (albeit someone else's) with all that this entailed, a presence that was expanded in the 1950s with the construction of the Distant Early Warning radar stations, or DEW-line. Secondly, the Mounties had two new programs to administer: the Eskimo disc system and the family allowances credits.

The disc system was introduced to make it easier for the white administration to identify the Inuit, to check relationships for family allowance entitlements, and so on. This was important because the Inuit did not have a system of family surnames and rarely spoke or wrote in English, while the white administrators rarely spoke Inuktitut. Consequently, Inuit names were often recorded incorrectly. Every Inuit was given a number, which was imprinted on a plastic disc that was usually worn around the neck or on the arm, like an army "dog tag." The whole of the Far North was divided into districts, which were identified by numbers: E1, E2, et cetera, through 9 in the east; and W1, W2, et cetera, through 9 in the west (see map 2). The individual numbers started with the number of the district in which the person lived and then were assigned in order of registration (for example, E7–123). The members of the same family usually had consecutive numbers, but of course this might not continue as new babies were born or children adopted.

Thus, the first inhabitants of Canada were again ahead of the rest of us – in being issued with identification numbers. Today, we all have social insurance numbers and usually need to carry them with us, though not, perhaps, around our necks. The disc system was in force until the late 1960s when, responding to pressure from both within and outside the Inuit community, the government replaced the number identification system with surnames chosen by the Inuit themselves.

The second program was the family allowances, or child credits, which applied to all of Canada. As the Inuit still had a mainly nonmonetary society, the RCMP were responsible for distributing the family allowances to them in the form of credits, at the local HBC store, for food or supplies (such as a rifle and ammunition to increase a family's natural food supply). Before they could do this, the Mounties had to register all the children and the adults responsible for them. In the process, they sometimes found that as many as 50 per cent of the children in a community had never had their births registered.

Naturally, in the North as elsewhere, some policemen were better than others. Their position encouraged them to be authoritarian, and the "distance" normally kept – at least, in those times – between figures of authority and the public may have translated into, or been seen as, prejudice or racism. Indeed, at times it may have been so. (One Inuk woman interviewed mentioned that on her birth certifi-

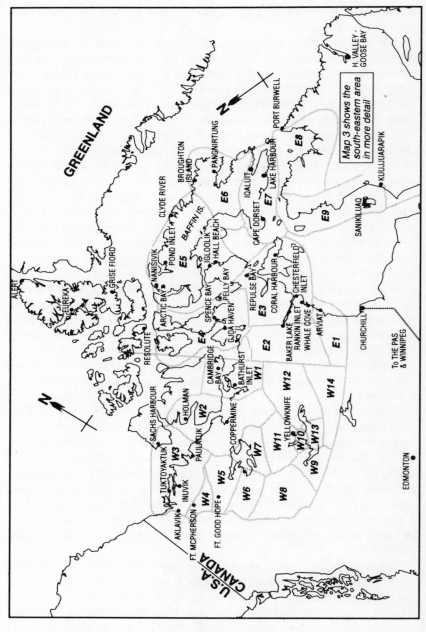

Map 2 Inuit Hamlets and Eskimo Registration Districts in the Northwest Territories (N.F. Fielding; Thames Label & Litho)

cate, issued by the local RCMP, her nationality was described as "Husky.")[12] But like the missionaries and traders, many of the RCMP officers spent long years in the North and learned the language and customs of the people. They may sometimes have felt that they were unfairly imposing southern laws and decisions on a people who lived in an entirely different frame of reference and had neither asked for these laws nor helped develop them; but as RCMP officers, they had been charged with enforcing the will of the government, and within their own terms of contract they probably did the best they could for the people. The RCMP appreciated the abilities of the Inuit and gave them the opportunity to get involved in the running of their communities as special constables.

As the programs to combat the TB epidemic began to be implemented, the RCMP played their part. They were primarily responsible for assembling the local Inuit for the medical surveys and patrols. Even if no overt coercion was used, the authority of their position and their accustomed role in the little communities probably helped to ensure compliance. In the 1950s they introduced radio-telephones into their detachments, and they were often the contact for news about relatives or returning evacuees; and they observed – and often vigorously and critically reported on – the way in which the people returned.

All the southern interlopers in the settlements had their specific roles to play. But in such isolated and hard conditions, the few whites had to cooperate with each other – their own emotional survival, if nothing else, depended on this – and there was probably a cross-influence of attitudes between all the players, just as there was neighbourly help in practical living.

PART TWO

The Events

CHAPTER FIVE

Emergence of the Problem

Isolation in their harsh climate preserved the Inuit from the ravages of southern diseases for thousands of years. But it also left them with no built up immunity, and when the Europeans began to arrive, inadvertently carrying the germs with them, epidemics of measles, influenza, poliomyelitis, and tuberculosis ravaged many of the communities. Usually, a disease hit one community or area, decimated the population, then retreated. But tuberculosis lingered, spread, and became endemic.

Several factors contributed to this. First, the severe cold (which has no effect on the tuberculosis bacillus) made the Inuit vulnerable to respiratory troubles and forced them to live in tiny, one-room dwellings for most of the year, so that an infectious disease such as tuberculosis almost inevitably spread from one infected person to the rest of the family. Second, as the Inuit adapted to accommodate the desires of the newcomers, trapping to exchange furs for store goods or working for the RCMP or on military construction sites for cash, their highly nutritious fresh-meat or fish diet and their warm caribou-skin clothing were gradually exchanged for a diet largely of white flour, lard, tea, jam, and canned goods, and for much less warm southern clothing. When the caribou declined or the pattern of migration changed (possibly as a result of the incursions of military and mining into the North), malnutrition occurred. This, combined with the inadequate clothing, increased the Inuit's vulnerability to the new diseases.

Hard information about the early stages of the epidemic is scanty, but a few suggestive remarks appear in the writings of people who visited or lived in the North. In 1861, for instance, C.F. Hall mentioned that consumption had killed more Inuit than all other diseases put together.[1] Another early reference to pulmonary diseases among the Inuit was by Lucien Turner in 1889 in a report for the American Bureau of Ethnology. Turner said that half of the Inuit in Kuujjuaq died of "pulmonary troubles," which proceeded at "an astonishing rate, soon carrying off the afflicted person."[2] Dr Wilfred Grenfell, after visiting five Moravian missions in Labrador in 1893, reported that he found a great deal of tuberculosis among the people.[3] Yet at the same time, reports coming from other areas of the Arctic often referred to the good health of the local population. So it would appear that until well into the twentieth century, tuberculosis did not have a hold on the population as a whole.

During the early part of this century, the attention of medical specialists in tuberculosis was concentrated on the southern population. Later, concern grew about the terrible situation among the native Indian population, and pressure from some doctors and the churches was directed towards dealing with the ravages of tuberculosis among them. For the Inuit, the need was at first simply to get them basic medical services of any sort. The missionaries, police, and traders provided some drugs and first aid, but they were not qualified to diagnose tuberculosis and were certainly in no position to treat it. Not until doctors went to the Arctic on a regular basis in the 1920s, either on the annual summer patrols or to work in the mission hospitals, did the tuberculosis situation begin to be recognized. But it seems that the officials of the Department of the Interior were loth to admit either that the situation was really serious or that they should – or could – do something about it. What happened at Coppermine is instructive.[4]

Dr R.D. Martin was appointed medical health officer at Coppermine, and in July 1929 he opened a medical station there to serve the important gathering place on the Coppermine River and an area of about 95 kilometres radius around it. Martin had a single-storey building of 9 by 5.5 metres as his combined home, surgery, and emergency ward, but no trained help or interpreter. Besides his medical duties, which included trips to outlying camps, he therefore had to supervise the untrained Inuit family he had hired to look after the patients and the little medical station, as well as handing out destitute rations when necessary, sending in reports on game and local conditions, and issuing mining licences.

When Martin arrived on the ship from Herschel Island, he found all the people to be healthy, though on the ship he had noticed three people with bone tuberculosis, two of them returning to the Coppermine district. Over the next 20 months he reported a marked increase in the incidence of tuberculosis. The first year, apart from the nearly universal bronchitis following the arrival of the ship, he dealt mainly with minor medical troubles. But he found cases of both pulmonary and bone tuberculosis scattered throughout the district. In one group of 150 who came into Coppermine, for instance, five had TB, of whom four died and one was improving in hospital 18 months later. Of twelve cases noted that year, nine died.

The next eight months showed a change from "sporadic and iso-lated cases of tuberculosis to the widespread and epidemic form," and "the effect of not isolating acutely infected cases" (for which he had no facilities) "was shown by ten deaths occurring in 3 families." In October that year (1930), Martin moved into a shack to provide additional room for patients. Meanwhile, he continued to treat people (many of whom refused to come to the hospital) in their tents or snow houses. Of these, 38 had TB (14 of them pulmonary, 9 miliary, 5 spinal, and the rest various); by March 1930, 26 had died and 8 were worse.

Martin appealed for help to his bosses at the Department of the Interior. He needed extra space for isolating patients, a trained orderly, and an interpreter to help persuade the people of the need to come into the hospital to prevent spreading the disease. But no help was forthcoming. Meanwhile, Bishop Breynat of the Roman Catholic church proposed to build a hospital at Coppermine and asked for a grant from the government. The mission wanted to build a two-storey structure in 1931–32. Martin favoured a smaller unit that could be put up quickly in 1931, to be run by the nondenomi-national government service. At one point, the 1931–32 Department of the Interior estimates included an item to cover a nurse and a grant for the proposed Roman Catholic hospital, but by February 1931 this item had been withdrawn. That month, the NWT council concluded that Martin's plans were "rather extensive" but that hos-pital facilities were needed at Coppermine and that this should again be brought to the attention of the minister.

In March 1931, Martin reported to the department, "Tuberculosis is present in every group in this area. In the Coppermine it reached epidemic proportions and out of about one hundred people, 22 died in 9 months, of whom 19 were tubercular, that is 25% per annum."[5] At the time, he thought that the epidemic was related to the minor infections brought in by passengers on the ship, which aggravated or lit up existing tubercular infections. Later, he ascribed it to the return home of one man who had been south and had there con-tracted TB of the hip, which became reactivated in the North, then became generalized and rapidly spread through the community. At the time of Martin's report there were still 15 known cases of tuberculosis in the district; he again detailed the additional modest facilities urgently required for isolating them, and also the need for an interpreter and an orderly.

Martin's appointment was terminated that summer of 1931, and the area was then covered by Dr J.A. Urquhart at Aklavik. In 1932, Urquhart similarly reported that the population was "infected with tuberculosis to a very marked extent,"[6] the majority of the cases being bone infections. But no hospital, either government or Catholic, was built at Coppermine, which had to wait until 1947 before it received even a nursing station.

Throughout the 1930s, most of the medical officers continued to report on the high incidence of TB in their areas and the need for better treatment services of one sort or another – all without any positive result. In 1934 Dr J.A. Bildfell in Pangnirtung wrote:

Tuberculosis is so general among Pangnirtung natives that to speculate on any particular percentage is impossible ... everything appears to be in favour of the germ, and nothing to the advantage of the native in combating the disease. It is the chief factor in ... the high child mortality rate [and] the main cause of death generally ... As far as Pangnirtung is concerned it so eclipses every other diseased condition that it might be said that there prevails but one disease among them. Thus the hospital should be equipped to treat tuberculosis as efficiently as possible.[7]

When the responsibility for Inuit health care passed to the new Department of Mines and Resources (DMR) in 1936 and the medical service came under Dr E.L. Stone, the reports and requests continued to come in. But the new department carried on the former policy – considering what to do, whether or not to establish sanatoria in the North, fending off criticism and suggestions, and certainly not increasing expenditures on medical services.

That year Dr A.G. Mackinnon reported from Pangnirtung, "The disease is so prevalent that the best one can hope for is to isolate the most dangerous spreaders,"[8] and Dr I.M. Rabinowitch on the Eastern Arctic Patrol reported that tuberculosis was common in the straits and bay. At Chesterfield Inlet, for instance, of the 62 people Rabinowitch examined, 12 had active tuberculosis, and at Port Burwell the proportion was 6 out of 31. At other settlements the rates were lower or the cases questionable; at some, no evidence of tuberculosis was found; and at others, such as Craig Harbour, the people were "exceptionally healthy."[9]

In 1937, Mackinnon was still reporting tuberculosis as the most important and prevalent malady in the Pangnirtung area,[10] and the Anglican mission wanted to expand the Pangnirtung hospital (which had beds for six general and two TB patients) to accommodate six more tubercular patients. But when the question of the establishment of sanatoria, which had long been the subject of investigations and reports, again came before the NWT council in May, Dr L.D. Livingstone opposed the extension. He maintained that for an area population of around 400 people, the existing accommodation was ample; that "Eskimos ... lived for long periods of time with a more or less dormant pulmonary tuberculosis"; and that "under our housing conditions, food and environment they did not survive for any length of time. Probably the most detrimental is the environment as a tubercular patient if he is not content, very rapidly declines."[11]

In the summer of 1938, Dr K.F. Rogers conducted a general medical survey of Inuit in the Eastern Arctic. While he gave a generally favourable report, he noted that his findings were not empirically based but were mainly a matter of opinion, and he recommended that a scientific study be carried out to get a clear picture of the situation. The government used this report, however, as the basis for stating that the Inuit population were in good health and (erroneously) that instances of tubercular disease among them were "less frequent than among whites."[12]

In August 1939, Dr T.J. Orford wrote to R.A. Gibson, director of the Bureau of Northwest Territories and Yukon Affairs at DMR, reporting TB as a major health problem and proposing the establishment of a model camp within four hours' sled or boat travel from Pangnirtung for "all cases whose treatment [after examination at the hospital] would be more satisfactory under improved living conditions and who are a source of infection to healthy natives in contact with them."[13] Orford seems to have envisaged a sort of halfway stage between hospital isolation and rehabilitation, where the selected families would live. They would continue to hunt or trap and live more or less their normal lives, but they would be out of contact with other camps, they would be under the weekly sanitary and medical supervision of the doctor, and would be supplied with good winter and summer tents, medicines, bedding, utensils, and supplementary nourishing food.[14] Nothing seems to have come from this suggestion either.

Outsiders also raised questions about the situation in the Arctic. An inquiry in 1939 from *Encyclopaedia Britannica* about "the health of Eskimos, with particular reference to tuberculosis" prompted a small flurry of activity in the bureau.[15] The Rev. Rokeby-Thomas, an Anglican missionary for five years in Cambridge Bay, had been reported in the *Daily Telegraph* as having told an Edmonton paper that tuberculosis was making severe inroads among the Inuit. Major

D.L. McKeand, superintendent of the Eastern Arctic and secretary of the NWT council, and for many years the main government representative on the Eastern Arctic Patrol, refuted this on the basis that in the Cambridge Bay–Coppermine area the birth rate had exceeded the death rate over the previous five years by 27 per cent. McKeand threw in the comment that "many requests for a resident doctor or at least a medical inspection, have come from Cambridge Bay in recent years. This area comes in for a good deal of publicity through Stefansson, Jenness and others of the Arctic Expedition of 1914–18, and until recently we found it difficult to prove that Baffin Island Eskimos were superior in health ... to those of the Queen Maud Gulf area. Since we moved them to Fort Ross and got the Police, the Hudson's Bay Company and the Missions to move their men from east to west, and vice versa, the question has been pretty well solved."[16]

Gibson referred the matter to Dr R. Millar at the Department of Pensions and National Health, who passed it to Dr G.J. Wherrett of the Canadian Tuberculosis Association. Wherrett's response provided the bulk of Gibson's subsequent reply to *Encyclopaedia Britannica*, namely, that the Inuit population was increasing and therefore either TB was not of epidemic proportions or it had passed the acute stage, probably the latter, but that it was in different stages in different Inuit camps; that it was present among the Inuit to a greater extent than among the white population; and that "the present arrangements for inspections and medical treatment ... are as satisfactory as can be effected, considering the terrain, the difficulties of travel and the many isolated, small groups of Eskimos."[17]

Nevertheless, pressure on the government to provide a better level of health care continued to grow. During World War II the U.S. forces came into the Canadian Arctic, setting up air bases, staging posts, and army hospitals for their Crimson Line evacuation route for the casualties anticipated in Europe, and they stayed on with the DEW-line bases after the war. By 1943, the physicians attached to the American bases were complaining about the "shocking ... condition of Inuit health and the medical care extended to them by the government of Canada," and returning airmen and construction workers began to describe the Inuit settlements they had visited in terms that reflected little credit on the administration.[18] In 1943 the Rockefeller Foundation sponsored a survey of conditions in the Canadian Arctic to be conducted by the Canadian Social Sciences and Research Council, and Wherrett was commissioned to survey health conditions and medical services in the Northwest Territories. His brief covered whites and Indians as well as Inuit, and he visited only the Mackenzie

River district, but he included statistical data from across the territories.

While Wherrett was compiling his data, personnel in the Department of Mines and Resources (DMR) continued to discuss the merits of the hospital policy in the Northwest Territories. A precis of the policy for the NWT council in June 1943 leaned heavily towards continuation of the current policy of subsidizing mission-owned hospitals. The grounds given were economy (the missionaries worked for nothing and raised money to help pay running costs so that government expenditures were minimal, and no capital costs were needed since no hospitals were under construction); adequacy (the doctors had full authority over nurses and the medical treatment of patients); and even civilizing effectiveness (the missionaries were brought into close contact with the natives, and hospitalization was synonymous with civilization and Christianity). The paper cited the average amount paid by the NWT administration to the mission hospitals during the previous three years, and the total for the four Arctic hospitals (supplying 109 beds) came to $25,550. This was for the day-to-day running costs of the hospitals and did not include the doctors' and nurses' salaries. The only advantages suggested if DMR took over the hospitals were that one of the two hospitals at Aklavik could then be closed, and that the doctors would have more say in the administration of the hospitals and DMR would have more say in deciding where any future ones would be located.[19]

In October 1943 Dr Livingstone, who had earlier opposed enlarging the hospital at Pangnirtung, urged the construction of a TB sanatorium at Fort McPherson to serve the Mackenzie Delta and Western Arctic as "one of the great needs in the Territories at the present time." He also suggested a sanatorium at Lake Harbour to serve the Eastern Arctic, and a third, smaller unit in the southern Northwest Territories.[20]

The same month an exchange of memos between Gibson and McKeand[21] revealed that "the pressing need for a resident medical officer at Fort Chimo [Kuujjuak had] been a live subject for the past decade"; and that the doctors at the Pangnirtung and Chesterfield hospitals refused admission to incurable tubercular Inuit and discharged terminally ill patients to die "in tents or snow houses," either because there were limited funds as a result of reduced appropriations or because they thought the prejudice of Inuit against going to hospital would increase if too many people died there. McKeand defended the wisdom of the resident doctors against the "itinerant, inexperienced" (in terms of the subarctic) doctors of the U.S. Army and on the Eastern Arctic Patrol ship, who had evidently criticized the treatment of the Inuit and who he doubted were "familiar with these well-known departmental regulations and practices." As he pointed out, "If ... there are unlimited funds available for the treatment of Eskimos, the hospitals at Pangnirtung and Chesterfield will welcome ... the chance to treat them, which has been practically denied to them heretofore." His parting shot was that "not one dollar of the provincial fur tax collected from Eskimos of the Ungava Bay area is available for their medical comfort."[22]

Gibson directed that the policy be reconsidered with Dr Millar, the medical assistant to the Department of Pensions and National Health, thus continuing the old practice of by-passing his own senior doctor. In February 1944, Millar wrote to Gibson praising DMR's system of medical treatment for northern natives, but suggesting again that three TB centres be set up in the North for open cases of tuberculosis, at Pangnirtung, Aklavik, and either Southampton Island or Chesterfield, because "the removal of northern natives to southern institutions is not good practice, but almost invariably the patients ... become lonesome, decline, and sometimes die." Millar advised that "the avoidance of removal of northern natives to southern institutions should be a stated principle as far as possible."[23]

In March 1944 Bishop Fleming, of the Anglican Diocese of the Arctic, wrote to Gibson inquiring about a hospital at Coppermine, where the local Anglican missionary was doing "an extraordinary amount of medical work," and suggesting that the department use army doctors and planes to expand the northern medical services. McKeand's memo for Gibson's response stressed the impossibility of persuading suitable doctors to work in the Arctic, the consequent vacancies at Chesterfield and Pangnirtung for the coming year, the unsuitability of the Eastern Arctic terrain for planes, and the detrimental effect that flights had on the wildlife on which the Inuit hunters depended.[24] The department did secure the services of some doctors seconded from the army, but this was in order to fill vacancies, not to expand the service.

Again, in the summer of 1944, Dr Falconer, reporting on his trip as medical officer to the Eastern Arctic Patrol (EAP), suggested that a TB sanatorium be set up at Kuujjuaq to serve the northern Quebec Inuit; or, if the local TB patients were to be flown out to southern sanatoria, that there should at least be a nursing station there. At that time there was a U.S. air base at Kuujjuaq that had a fully equipped 100-bed hospital, with operating rooms, x-ray, dental facilities, and so on, and the medical unit provided some medical and dental treatment for the local Inuit, some of whom worked at the base. Falconer seems to have assumed that the department could acquire some of this equipment after the war to set up a more modest sanatorium.[25]

Falconer would have had a very busy time in the Ungava Bay area had all the Inuit been in the settlements when he visited in June–July. In January, McKeand had sent a memo to Gibson listing the reasons why the EAP should call at Kuujjuaq. These included the "medical examination of approximately 257 Eskimos and 192 Indians" and the "medical examination of sick Eskimos from George River [Kangiqsualujjuaq] and Payne Bay [Kangirsuk] (approximately 548 people)". McKeand concluded that "the maximum of 48 hours would be all the time that could be spared for the inspection."[26] In the event, Falconer went by plane and spent two days in Kuujjuaq, where he found 100 Inuit, very little illness, and a great deal of help from the U.S. base's doctor and dentist. At Kangirsuk, where he spent another day, only 30 Inuit were in camp, and at Kangiqsualujjuaq only four. So he was able to check only 134 of the 805 Inuit in the district. Fortunately, the bulk of the group were receiving medical attention from the resident U.S. doctors. A nursing station was eventually set up at Kuujjuaq in 1949.

The year 1945 was crucial in the development of the anti-TB campaign in the North. In January the government set up an Advisory Committee for the Control and Prevention of Tuberculosis among Indians, which was given "the authority ... to inquire into the present methods of tuberculosis prevention, detection, treatment and aftercare ... of Indians"[27] and the responsibility to report to government with a view to "correlating (all governmental) anti-tuberculosis work ... and (recommending) the best possible use of monies ... for the purpose of eradicating and preventing the spread of the disease among Indians".[28] Although the committee's terms of reference specified Indians, it was to have a great influence on the tuberculosis program that was eventually set up for the Inuit. The committee stemmed from a proposal made in 1937 by Dr Wherrett and the Canadian Tuberculosis Association (CTA) to undertake a study of the tuberculosis problem; this had led to a conference that year with representatives drawn exclusively from the medical profession, from the federal and provincial ministries, the CTA, the sanatoria, and specialists in the disease. As P.G. Nixon has pointed out, the "view which developed from this conference was that tuberculosis was essentially a medical, as opposed to a broader social-economic, phenomena and therefore was to be solved, if at all, by medical practitioners."[29]

The 1945 advisory committee was also virtually limited to the medical profession. It consisted of twelve members, "ten of who, including the chairman, shall be nominated by the Department of Health and Welfare (Dr Brock Chisholm, the Deputy Minister was their first nominee), and one to be a senior medical officer of the Indian Affairs Branch of the Department of Mines and Resources, who shall act as secretary of the committee."[30] Dr P.E. Moore, who had taken over the directorship of the Indian Health Services when Stone returned to the army at the outbreak of World War II, was DMR's first representative on the committee.[31]

In February 1945, Wherrett's report on his Mackenzie Delta survey was published. It provided the first authoritative estimate of tuberculosis among the Inuit.[32] Wherrett's views seem to have changed since 1939, when he felt the service to be "as satisfactory as can be effected." He identified the particular health problems of the Inuit as (1) tuberculosis, with a death-rate for Inuit of 314 per 100,000 population compared with 53 per 100,000 for the rest of Canada; (2) pneumonia (203 per 100,000 compared with 52); and (3) diseases of the first year (166 compared with 54). He also reported a very large proportion of ill-defined or unknown causes of death for the Inuit population (740 per 100,000, as opposed to 44 for the white population of the Northwest Territories), these being the 84 per cent of Inuit deaths that took place without a doctor or nurse being available. He thought that this group probably included many deaths from tuberculosis, so even the official high death rate from this disease was probably an underestimate. Wherrett concluded that the problem was staggering.

While praising the efforts of the few lone doctors and nurses, the missionaries, the RCMP, the traders and their wives, and the native people themselves, for their courage and devotion in attempting to give medical care to the sick, Wherrett was fiercely critical of government, and he made several suggestions for improvement. As far as tuberculosis was concerned, he called for:

1 the construction of a sanatorium at Fort Smith, to be operated by the government and be the headquarters for a TB officer and an annual diagnostic x-ray service visiting all centres;
2 better use of existing hospital beds (e.g., at Aklavik) for treatment of TB; he found 150 empty beds that could be used for this purpose if the hospitals were brought up to standard with adequate funding, operating, laboratory, and x-ray facilities, and with decisions for admissions, etc., put into the hands of the medical officers;
3 a medical airplane service for emergencies and regular visits by medical officers to outlying settlements;

4 x-ray examinations, vaccinations, immunizations, and the evacuation of active cases of tuberculosis from all the schools (mainly
Indian mission schools).[33]

Wherrett also suggested that there be additional qualified medical
officers, nursing stations, and dental services; a reorganized, inte-
grated medical service, in which the doctors would be free of such
additional government functions as serving as the local Indian agent;
and nutritional studies and surveys of the population. Wherrett's
report probably put the final seal on the realization that the problem
of tuberculosis among the Inuit had to be addressed in a more
effective way. With the advisory committee, the medical profession
had at last moved into the driver's seat, and the responsibility for
medical care for all native peoples, Indian and Inuit, was about to be
turned over to the new Department of National Health and Welfare.

The changeover took place on 1 November 1945, and that fall and
winter the NWT administration summarized its current arrangements
for the medical care of the Inuit[34] and sent the new deputy minister
of health and welfare its suggestions on "Planning Medical Care of
Eskimo," in which additional hospitals or sanatoria were again proposed for Coppermine, Moffet Inlet, Lake Harbour, Cape Dorset,
Inukjuak, and Kuujjuaq.[35] But from these documents it appears that
despite all the protests, suggestions, and memos, there had been no
improvement in the situation since 1939, and there had probably
been a deterioration. The cost of medical care, covering salaries of
medical staff, medical supplies, and hospitalization, had risen by
only $2,315 to a total of $47,795 ($29,021 for running costs, $18,774
for salaries), or $6.46 per person (using the 1941 census figures). Of
this sum, $19,174 was spent in the Western Arctic, where 1,392 Inuit
were living in 1941, for a rate of $13.77 per person – perhaps not too
bad. But in the Eastern Arctic, where 80 per cent of the population,
or 6,000 people lived, only $28,620 was spent, amounting to the
princely sum of $4.77 for each person. And despite all the discussions
and proposals during the 15 years since the Coppermine episode, no
additional medical staff or new facilities – sanatoria, hospitals, or
nursing stations – had been provided for the Arctic. It was a sorry
record.

CHAPTER SIX

The Assault

Having wrested control of Inuit health care from the Department of Mines and Resources, Dr Moore and his colleagues in the Indian Health Service (IHS) launched their attack on tuberculosis. The Inuit and tuberculosis were not, of course, their only concerns. Health services for Indians were also their responsibility, and this represented an enormous challenge because the Indians also had a very high incidence of tuberculosis and had suffered from the same chronic underfunding of medical services as the Inuit. But the timely combination of the end of the war and the consequent freeing-up of money and medical personnel from the forces, the switch in departmental authority, Wherrett's report, and the fact that a parliamentary committee had just been set up to revise the Indian Act, helped to persuade Parliament to vote a large increase in the budget of the new department. This allowed it scope for really effective treatment programs.

The initial plans were simple if extensive: survey the whole population with x-rays to discover the active cases; remove these people from the community to lessen the spread of the disease, preferably sending them to southern sanatoria for active treatment; and immunize as many of the rest of the population as practicable with BCG vaccine. Refinements to the plan were made over the years, but this approach remained the heart of IHS strategy through the 1960s.

In the east, the x-ray surveys got off to a quick start but then ran into trouble. The first summer of the new regime, an enlarged medical team, which included a dentist, an eye surgeon, and an x-ray technician and x-ray equipment, was sent with the Eastern Arctic Patrol on the HBC supply ship *Nascopie*. Some 1,500 Inuit were x-rayed,[1] although the films had to be taken back to Ottawa for interpretation, and consequently active cases were left in the communities for another year. The next year, 1947, the *Nascopie* was sunk on a rock off Cape Dorset, and the government had to scramble to get planes and small ships to complete the work of the patrol.[2] Both the USAF and the RCAF helped, and 42 people who had been x-rayed the previous summer were flown out for treatment.[3]

The patrol was similarly handicapped in 1948 and 1949,[4] but in 1950 the new coastguard ship *C.D. Howe* was in commission and the surveys were resumed, with more than 1,000 x-rays that year.[5] The medical team did more than just take x-rays. They also made a quick medical examination of each person in the settlements at which they called, vaccinated or inoculated the people against various diseases such as measles and whooping-cough, did some dental work and medical treatment, consulted with the nurse if there was one or with her proxy if there was not, left medical supplies, and decided which people should be evacuated for treatment elsewhere. Life and procedures on the *C.D. Howe* are described in the next chapter, but the following figures give some idea of the scope of the early surveys carried out from this ship:

1954:   931 x-rays;
1955:   1,500 x-rays, 105 people evacuated;
1956:   saturation survey of the east coast of Baffin;
1957:   1,394 people surveyed, 93 evacuated.[6]

The IHS also made use of any doctors who were in Inuit territory, particularly in the east, including those at the USAF bases at Southampton Island, Iqaluit and Kuujjuaq. In 1946 the doctor at the Catholic mission hospital at Chesterfield, Major Rawson, who had been seconded from the RCAMC, mentioned in his report on the death of six people from TB on Southampton Island that x-rays of 64 persons and sputum from 14 had been taken by the U.S. medical officer at the base on Southampton Island and had been passed to the *Nascopie* or the RCMP the previous summer for analysis. (No replies had yet been received.) The U.S. army hospital had also treated some patients and had performed an autopsy on at least one of the dead.[7] In the same period, 1945–46, the medical officer to the Canadian forces carrying out Exercise Musk-Ox in the area north of Churchill was asked to x-ray (using a portable unit) as many Inuit as possible wherever he set up medical stations at the various outposts along the line of march.[8] And in July 1948 a group from Queen's University was in the same Keewatin–Southampton Island area taking x-rays.

The first major survey involving Western Arctic Inuit was carried out in April 1949 by Dr Callaghan from Aklavik. He took portable x-ray equipment and some medical supplies and vaccines to the trading posts between Aklavik and Spence Bay, starting from Norman Wells in a chartered Canadian Pacific Airlines single-engine Norseman. His party consisted of just a handful of people: the CPA pilot, Ernie Boffa; a mechanic, Glen McKinnon; and an intelligence officer from Western Command, Major Douthewaite. All of them helped the doctor in both the x-raying and the immunization procedures. They were also helped at each stop by some of the local residents. Callaghan's report gives a good picture of the work performed by the field doctors and the conditions with which the early western surveys had to contend.[9]

Callaghan and his party left Norman Wells on 17 April, called in at Fort Norman to arrange to leave the exposed film to be developed there at the end of the survey, then flew on to Coppermine. Here they stayed one night, x-rayed and vaccinated 206 people, and treated a few minor problems before flying off to the next post at Burnside Harbour. At Burnside they stayed two nights and surveyed 148 people before going on to Cambridge Bay. Here they discovered an epidemic of influenza pneumonia, and Callaghan had to take emergency action. He set up a five-ward emergency hospital with the help of the RCAF station, started the patients on penicillin, and made two sorties to out-camps, where people were reported to be sick, and evacuated one camp. Finally, he arranged for a doctor and two nurses to fly in from Edmonton before the team left to continue the survey.

They ran into many problems. Often, they had difficulty finding their way over the featureless terrain or in poor visibility, with the compass "useless ... being so close to the magnetic north pole." The pilot had to land between posts several times to check his maps – even, on one occasion, to ask a man with a dog team exactly where they were. In one tiny settlement their x-ray motor was frozen overnight. They arrived at one post to find no Inuit there, for the people had not been alerted to the survey, but in other camps they were often x-raying until midnight and then were away at seven o'clock next morning. They had to sit out bad weather – and sometimes flew into it so unexpectedly that only the pilot's promptitude and knowledge of the terrain saved them from a crash. Nevertheless, they arrived safely back at Aklavik on 1 May, having called at Coppermine, Burnside, Cambridge Bay, Perry River, Sherman Inlet, Gjoa Haven, Spence, Read Island, Holman Island, and Stanton. In just two weeks they had travelled well over 3,000 kilometres, had x-rayed and immunized 791 Inuit, discovered and dealt with the influenza pneumonia epidemic at Cambridge Bay, and along the way had treated sundry people who required medical attention.

By Christmas 1949, Dr Moore was congratulating his staff on their achievements to date. In the IHS director's newsletter he wrote: "The year just closing has been a very active one, and we can all look upon it as a year of achievement. Possibly the major accomplishment of the year was the widespread x-ray surveys from the Gulf of St. Lawrence to the islands of the Pacific where active, well-planned x-ray surveys were carried out."[10] These surveys, of course, applied to the Indian clientele of the IHS as well as the Inuit.

In 1950 only small surveys were done in the west, both of them in April. One was from Aklavik, examining the 45 Inuit employed on a project to re-establish the caribou herd, and the other was from Cambridge Bay in which 97 people were seen. A major survey was carried out in the east in addition to that done on the *C.D. Howe*. From June to September a party headed by Dr R.N. Simpson and including a dentist and a technician travelled the James Bay catchment area of the new Moose Factory hospital, x-raying 2,419 Indians, 850 Inuit, and 205 white residents.[11]

From 1951 on, the western surveys were mainly organized from the Charles Camsell Hospital in Edmonton. They included x-ray technicians on the team and were carried out in the spring by air. The first major western survey, at Easter 1953, drew on information provided by Callaghan's report of 1949 and by a relatively unsuccessful survey conducted in 1951 via a Hudson's Bay Company supply schooner that had sailed along the coast during the summer when most of the people were away hunting.[12] In the 1953 survey, 927 Inuit and 25 whites were x-rayed from a base set up at Cambridge Bay, where the RCAF had its winter survival school. A ski-equipped Norseman was again used to fly into the smaller communities, but the patients were collected for evacuation at Cambridge Bay. From there, they were flown south in the large RCAF transport planes. For many years, this remained the main route to the sanatorium for the Western Arctic Inuit. Don Harkness, the technician then in charge of the Charles Camsell x-ray department, described the conditions under which the survey team worked:

The survey was carried out under severe stress and hardship. There were no hotels or restaurants at that time, nor suitable facilities in which to do the survey. The X-ray crew slept in sleeping bags on the floor of either the church or the Hudson's Bay store which is where they also set up their equipment. They cooked their own food which had been brought with them. In carrying out the survey they had to improvise at every site. To develop X-ray films it was necessary to create a darkroom, melt the snow for water and heat it to the proper temperature. Films were developed on site in order to make an immediate provisional diagnosis which would enable people with suspected active TB to be congregated at Cambridge Bay then evacuated by the RCAF to Edmonton.[13]

What happened at the holding station at Cambridge Bay was described by Kathleen Dier, who opened the nursing station there for Health and Welfare in 1956:

At one time we had 14 active TB patients living in the nursing station awaiting transportation to Edmonton. Gwen [her Inuk nursing-aide/interpreter] and I tried to set up a system of separate dishes and we kept a pot of caribou stew on the stove for them while Pete [her local handyman] made bannock. The patients slept in sleeping bags on the floor and Gwen and I had our double bunk in the bedroom, occasionally shared with babies who would not stop crying until we took them into the security of our sleeping bags. They were so used to being in their mothers' parkas that the sudden wrench into the outside world was terrifying.[14]

The DEW-line station some 6 kilometres away sent its Bombardier over to pick up the sick and take them to the landing strip.

Getting the patients sent off to Camsell was an operation of military proportions; everyone had to be ready to board the RCAF flying boxcar the minute it landed on the ice. Each person had a big yellow tag with name, disc number and other particulars filled in at the top and bottom. The bottom part was removed at the Yellowknife hospital where the patients spent the night. The remainder was supposed to remain in place until they reached Camsell, a feat not usually accomplished as the wind kept blowing them away. This of course caused great confusion on their arrival at Camsell, confusion compounded by the fact that in fur parkas it wasn't easy to even sort out the men from the women. For the Inuit the trip south was a bewildering experience but they coped amazingly well.[15]

During the spring surveys, the RCAF transported most patients from the Western Arctic between Cambridge Bay, Yellowknife, and Edmonton. They used Hercules cargo planes, with a bench or bucket seats along one side for the passengers. At other times of the year, individual patients might be taken to Aklavik to catch the regular, though infrequent, air service to Edmonton. Local transport to and from Cambridge Bay or Aklavik was usually in the hands of the bush

Table 6
Early Inuit X-ray Survey and Hospitalization Figures

Year	No. of x-rays	No. of hospital admissions[1]	Total no. under care	No. in hospital on 31 December
1953	–	376	686	348
1954	5,210	420	768	406[2]
1955	7,188	950	1,356	698
1956	–	870	1,568[3]	703
1957	6,459	583	1,286	535
1958	7,462	547	1,082	450
1959	6,765	490	940	345
1960	9,512	448	793	295

Sources: Department of National Health and Welfare, IHS and INHS annual reports, 1954–60; G.J. Wherrett, *The Miracle of the Empty Beds* (Toronto: University of Toronto Press 1977) and *Tuberculosis in Canada* (Ottawa: Royal Commission on Health Services 1965).

[1] Includes first admissions, readmissions, and transfers.

[2] IHS annual report, 1956. (Wherrett gives 344 here.)

[3] Jenness (*Eskimo Administration*, vol. 2) and Robertson (*The Future of the North*) quote 1,578 here.

pilots or the RCMP. They flew small planes, such as the Norseman, which could land in the small posts in all kinds of weather and sometimes under hazardous conditions. These planes were a vital part of the early TB evacuation.

The spring and summer x-ray survey programs across the Arctic continued through the 1950s. By 1955 it was estimated that about 5,000 Inuit, or half the population, had been x-rayed, some of them more than once. And the numbers evacuated south steadily grew until in 1956 approximately one out of every seven Inuit was in a sanatorium in the south.[16] Table 6 shows the progression through the 1950s.

Where did all these Inuit patients go? Even before the new department was in operation, Dr Moore had been negotiating with the Department of National Defence (DND) to acquire some of its surplus hospitals to use for his Indian patients. One of these was the Jesuit College Hospital in Edmonton. This establishment had been built as a college in 1913, bought by the government in 1942, and handed over to the U.S. Army as a base of operations for the construction of the Alaska Highway. When the highway was finished in 1944, the Americans passed it back, much enlarged with temporary redwood buildings. DND then renovated and extended the complex into "a modern, fully equipped, 400 bed hospital with necessary appurtenances." By July 1945, however, the hospital had only 22 patients, and by the end of the year the government had been persuaded to transfer it to Health and Welfare for the Indian Health Service (IHS). Slightly redesigned to accommodate 350 tuberculous, medical, and surgical cases, the hospital was formally opened in August 1946 and named the Charles Camsell Indian Hospital after the retiring deputy minister of mines and resources.[17] It became the main sanatorium to which Inuit from the Western Arctic were sent. Also acquired by 1947 were the U.S. Army hospital Clearwater Lake at The Pas (with 175 beds) and the Brandon Sanatorium (200 beds), an ex-DND hospital. Both hospitals were converted to be used exclusively for tuberculosis and were operated for the IHS by the Sanatorium Board of Manitoba.[18]

Edmonton was the regional headquarters for the Indian Health Service, and the Camsell staff became the main group organizing and carrying out the x-ray surveys in Alberta, the western part of the territories, and the Western Arctic. They also took on the bulk of the interpretation of x-rays taken in the field and assumed a supervisory role over tuberculosis treatment in the small mission hospitals in the western territories; these included the two mission hospitals at Aklavik and a later one at Fort Smith to which some Inuit were sent.

Winnipeg became the IHS administrative centre for the central Arctic and the Keewatin, from which patients were sent to the Clearwater Lake or Brandon sanatoria, or to a number of hospitals in Manitoba and Saskatchewan. Ottawa was the location both of the headquarters of the IHS and the administration of the Eastern Arctic and the northern Quebec regions. Patients from the east were initially scattered throughout the Maritimes, Ontario, and Quebec (particularly at Parc Savard, the Quebec Immigration Hospital), but were later concentrated mainly at the Mountain Sanatorium in Hamilton or at Weston in Toronto.

In 1948 the IHS began construction on a 165-bed hospital at Moose Factory, Ontario, at the foot of James Bay, to serve both Indians and Inuit from the bay area in northern Ontario and from the Quebec coast as far north as Salluit. For administrative purposes, the Ungava Bay area of northern Quebec farther round the coast was attached to Labrador, although the medical services for the area continued to be handled by the IHS. Labrador itself was still serviced by the International Grenfell Association. Moose Factory opened in September 1950 under considerable staffing difficulties (severe shortage and high turnover) and hampered by lack of accommodation for staff families, virtually no occupational programs for the patients, and an unhappy mix of two-thirds Indian and one-third Inuit patients who did not get along too well together.[19]

The IHS rejected continued suggestions from the Department of Mines and Resources (and even from some of its own doctors, for instance the medical officer on the 1948 Eastern Arctic Patrol) to build a TB sanatorium in the Arctic. In April 1948, Dr Falconer, the assistant director, wrote to R.A. Gibson, deputy commissioner of the Northwest Territories, that "we do not contemplate building a hospital in the NWT for the treatment of tuberculosis. As the surveys reveal cases requiring treatment and as beds are available at Edmonton, patients will be shipped to Edmonton."[20] Falconer also mentioned that the small mission hospitals had been underused in the past and that although they were far from ideal for the active treatment of tuberculosis, the IHS considered it advisable to use them to capacity before further building was done.

The arguments usually put forward for refusing to provide sanatoria treatment in the North were, first, that it was not possible to attract specialists to the region and that adequate modern treatment was therefore not possible; second, that the number of active TB cases was expected to decline within five years, so extra beds in the North would then be superfluous; and, third, that the main purpose of hospitalization in the North was not so much to give active treatment as to remove the infection source from the community, which could be done using the present facilities.[21]

During 1948 the NWT council asked the IHS to undertake the medical and hospital care for the rest of the residents for whom the NWT administration had previously been responsible. The service was happy to do this. It was less happy, however, when some of these people arrived at the Camsell hospital expecting to receive free treatment and travelling expenses like those provided for Indian and Inuit patients; and in December, Moore sent a circular letter to his field medical officers spelling out the policy of the service regarding treatment at this hospital. More specifically, Moore's circular provides a clear statement of his policy regarding the hospitalization of the Indians and Inuit who were his prime responsibility:

The main purpose of the [Charles Camsell] hospital is to treat tuberculosis in Indians and Eskimos who are wards of the Government. Beds in the hospital at present are at a premium and to take advantage of the facilities provided, priority should be given to patients whose condition is such that they are likely to improve with specialist treatment. A far advanced case with no hope of recovery might well be cared for at the hospital nearest to the home of the patient. A hopeless case may well be isolated in the home of the patient.

While it may be argued that hospitals in the N.W.T. are not suitable to care for active (bacillary) cases, it is known that in some of the hospitals, facilities are available, and little change would be necessary to maintain a proper technique of segregation and treatment.[22]

Moore used financial arguments to support his policy. Prior to the takeover of the IHS by Health and Welfare, the government paid mission hospitals $2.50 per patient day, but the mission hospitals at Pangnirtung and Chesterfield also received a grant for nurses' salaries and for the transportation of coal, which brought their actual subsidies to close to $5.00 a day. This compared with a sum of between $2.50 and $3.00 a day paid to southern institutions. By the end of the war, the missions found that their costs had risen so much that the amount they received from the government did not cover their expenses and they had to supplement their income by fundraising activities to keep the hospitals afloat. They therefore asked the government for more money.[23] From April 1947, Moore changed the basis of payment to a flat amount per patient day of $7.00, but with no additional subsidies. He thereafter pointed out that hospital costs were much more expensive in the Northwest Territories (for example, the new Yellowknife Hospital was charging $10 a day) than they were in the South, where costs were running at an average of $4.27 a day. This was a sizable factor in favour of long-stay sanatorium treatment in the South, and Moore maintained that it more than balanced the cost of transport south.

But with the new emphasis on hospitalization, even the mission hospitals – at least, those in Aklavik – soon found themselves more than full. Dr Schaefer said that in the mid-1950s, when he worked there, the Roman Catholic hospital "was always crowding patients in everywhere" so that the average patient population was more than double the number of beds available by southern standards, and that "70 to 80 per cent of the patient population consisted of tuberculous patients."[24] Thus, the mission hospitals were probably able to cover their costs, though they were never able to upgrade their facilities so that they could treat active cases in the way the IHS required.

Moore also used the higher success rates in the southern sanatoria as an argument against further support or expansion of the mission hospitals in the North. At a 1954 meeting of the Eskimo Advisory Committee, for instance, he cited the ratio of deaths to discharges in the northern hospitals as 29 per cent, compared with 13 per cent in hospitals in the South. This convinced the commissioner of the RCMP, for one, to support Moore's point of view.[25] Of course, by selecting the patients who would best respond to treatment to be evacuated south while leaving those "with no hope of recovery" in the North, Moore had arranged the comparative results that the IHS achieved. Whatever the merits of this policy from a medical or a compassionate point of view, it seems hardly fair to have used its predetermined results as a stick with which to beat the mission hospitals.

In the early days of the southern hospitalization program, Inuit requiring hospital treatment, whether for TB or for some other cause, were sent, in the words of one doctor, to wherever there happened to be a bed vacant. Only in New Brunswick, Prince Edward Island, and British Columbia were there no Inuit patients. Those who went to the larger centres, such as the Charles Camsell or Parc Savard or, later, the Mountain Sanatorium, were the lucky ones. In some of the hospitals there might be only one or two Inuit patients; and however good the medical treatment was, their isolation, lack of money, different language, and great difficulty in communicating either with their families or with those around them (or in taking advantage of whatever occupational facilities were available for other patients) increased their loneliness and homesickness; and made recovery more uncertain and slow.

Sometimes, not even the IHS knew where all the hospitalized Inuit were or could produce accurate identifying information about them. Until 1950, the Department of Mines and Resources (DMR) was responsible for all other aspects of Inuit administration, and by 1949 DMR officials were receiving anxious inquiries about people who had been brought out for treatment but about whom no reports had been received, either by their relatives or by the officials (who had, in fact, lost control over the movements of "their" population). They therefore developed a card-index system to chart the movement of Inuit to and between hospitals in the South, and sent off the first of many requests to the IHS, asking for a list of the Inuit in hospital and details of the sanatoria they were in, the date of admission, and a progress report. They also suggested that in future a semi-yearly or yearly report should be sent to the relatives with a copy to DMR.[26]

Moore agreed to this, and in February 1950 the first nominal roll of Inuit patients was sent to the department, which had been reorganized and was now called Resources and Development (DRD). This list showed that there were 119 patients, not all of them tubercular, scattered in 17 hospitals in the Northwest Territories, Manitoba, Nova Scotia, Ontario, and Quebec, and one patient whose hospital was not given. Some patient identification details (home location, disc number) of 42 of these people were either omitted or incomplete, or wrong. A DRD summary list for October 1950 gave a total of 129 Inuit in 11 hospitals outside the Northwest Territories and five for whom the hospital was unknown.[27]

As the hospitalization program picked up steam, complaints came in from all sides, particularly from the RCMP and the missionaries, about the lack of reports on patients, the tardy return of many of them, and the extreme unhappiness of both the relatives and the patients.[28] In 1951, G.E.B. Sinclair of DRD told Moore that the list of patients in Winnipeg and Brandon provided by Health and Welfare in Ottawa did not correspond with those identified by Dr Wood, the regional superintendent in Winnipeg. Sinclair complained that they had great difficulty in getting accurate and up-to-date information on Inuit patients and that this made both the rehabilitation of the patients and relations with the settlements very difficult. In 1952 Leo Manning from DRD began visiting the Inuit in hospital and suggesting the transfer, if possible, of lonely patients to hospitals where there was a larger group of Inuit. The nominal roll for December 1952 showed 207 people in 19 hospitals and two in "unknown" locations. The personal identification of 18 patients was incomplete.[29]

In 1953 the department was reorganized yet again and renamed Northern Affairs and National Resources (NANR), though the branch administering Inuit affairs remained essentially the same. An NANR summary for June 1953 giving the numbers of Inuit patients outside the Northwest Territories showed 264 in 9 hospitals, with no "unknown" designations.[30] A later NANR study on Inuit TB discharges listed 35 hospitals as treating Inuit for TB in 1954, giving the number of patients discharged from hospital during the year as 288.[31] Table 7 summarizes the lists for 1950–53.

In 1953 the IHS noted in its newsletter a big jump in the number of people (who may have been either Indian or Inuit) who, inexplicably, were refusing TB treatment (84 in 1952, 158 in 1953).

In 1954 things came to a head. The officer in charge of the Eastern Arctic Patrol for NANR was an ex-naval officer, B.G. Sivertz, and the ship was carrying several journalists and academics as passengers on various assignments. After the trip, Sivertz put in a scathing report not only about the conduct of the ship but also about the conduct of some of the crew and the medical contingent; and one of the journalists wrote a highly critical article on the same subject, which appeared in the *Vancouver Sun* in September.[32] In November, Donald Marsh, the Anglican bishop of the Arctic, stepped into the fray. He had continued to press for more hospitals, both through the Eskimo Affairs Committee and in direct talks with Moore and his colleagues, and when he realized he was getting nowhere he wrote directly to the prime minister, Louis St Laurent, about the way the Inuit were being treated.

Bishop Marsh wanted the southern hospitalization program – and the hardship he believed it caused the Inuit – to be replaced by the establishment of more hospitals in the Arctic. He said that on his Arctic trip that year he had heard "that the Eskimos fled inland

Table 7
Record of Inuit in Hospital, 1950–53

Hospital	Feb. 1950 IHS nominal roll	Oct. 1950 DRD summary	Dec. 1952 IHS nominal roll	June 1953 NANR summary
NORTHWEST TERRITORIES				
Aklavik RC	14	n/a	–	n/a
Aklavik Ang.	33	n/a	–	n/a
Chesterfield Inlet	16	n/a	1	n/a
Pangnirtung	8	n/a	1	n/a
NOVA SCOTIA				
RCN, Halifax	–	12	2	–
Dartmouth	1	–	1	–
Dartmouth Mental	1	–	–	–
NEWFOUNDLAND				
RCAF Goose Bay	–	3	–	–
QUEBEC				
Parc Savard	11	26	84	102
Sacré Coeur, Cartierville	–	–	1	–
St Michael's Roberval	–	–	1	–
Montreal General	–	} 3	–	–
Ste-Justine, Montreal	–		1	–
Sacred Heart, Caughnawaga	–	–	15	–
ONTARIO				
Essex Co. San.	1	–	–	–
Moose Factory	–	5	–	–
Ste-Thérèse, Moosonee	1	–	–	–
Mountain San.	–	–	4	8
Sunnybrook	–	1	–	–
Weston San.	1	1	6	5
MANITOBA				
Brandon San.	6	} 14	7	7
Brandon Mental	4		3	–
The Pas	–	–	–	4
Clearwater Lake	3	2	4	4
Dynevor, Selkirk	–	–	–	1
Selkirk Mental	1	1	2	–
Provincial Mental	–	–	1	–
St Boniface	1	–	5	3
King George, Winnipeg	–	} 19	–	–
Winnipeg Municipal	16		–	–
ALBERTA				
Charles Camsell	–	42	65	130
Provincial Mental	–	–	3	–
Hospital Unknown	1	5	2	–
Totals	119	134	209	264
Personal identification incomplete[1]	42	n/a	18	n/a

Source: National Archives of Canada, RG85, vols. 1129–252-3(2), 1129-252-3(3), and 1475-252-4(1).
[1] No home location, no disc number, or disc number wrong or incomplete.

before the arrival of the ship with the medical officers on board, for fear that they would be wrested from their homes and shipped outside never to return, as has happened to so many of their friends and relatives. It is indeed hard to believe that this is the only way that a great nation like Canada can care for a small minority in her midst and who are, after all, our oldest Canadians."[33] He enclosed his "Cry the Beloved Eskimo," a collection of "simple stories, all of which I can personally vouch for as true," to illustrate his concerns. The following are three of his stories.

1

The pale, reflected light of an Arctic night showed the dark shape of the landing barge as it chugged toward shore. In the harbour a mile or so away the lights of the anchored ship cast a beam of light across the waters ... A policeman stepped ashore, called out six names, and said he wanted them immediately. No one moved. Again he called out, and at last little groups slowly made their way from one tent to another. "Hurry! The tide is dropping and the ship sails almost at once," the Law called out.

Amid stunned silence two or three of those commanded to go woodenly picked up tobacco, matches, a Bible and a prayer book and obediently went to the boat. One poor old woman could not walk; she had to be almost carried. There was no time for farewells to children or relatives out visiting. The policeman's command was imperative. Again he commanded the two others to appear. At last, after repeated calls by relatives, someone discovered the missing people had gone off into the hills behind the settlement, rather than go to the white man's land on the boat. To them, as to many others, all too vivid were their memories of one of the tribe who had been commanded to get on an airplane one autumn, and of whom nothing had been heard for more than a year. Many others had gone out and not come back, and it had been years since they had left. The scow pulled out to the ship without a word being spoken. The four faced the unknown.

Up the ship's ladder they climbed until they reached the little knot of people standing above. The third person was a woman who, on arriving at the top, tossed back her hood to disclose the small baby in her pouch. The doctor, a tall white man, spotted it immediately. "Take that baby out and give it to another woman in the tender!" The mother protested, but to no avail. Someone whisked the child from her hood and thrust it into the arms of another woman who was without even a pouch on her parka for the child. The sobbing figure of the mother was hustled below and the unwilling foster mother thrust into a waiting boat. The telegraph rang. The ship sailed.

Was this the Soviet Union? No. Arctic Canada.

2

The missionary travelling on the ship went ashore to visit. Here were Eskimos, people amongst whom he had worked for a year, people he loved. The tent was new and across its width was a sleeping bench built of stones and wood, covered with a willow mat and skins. The housewife sat sewing socks. She threw them down and welcomed the visitor as he entered. *He* came from the outside, the white man's land, and therefore *He* would know the answer.

"Have you seen my daughter?" she begged. "My little four-year-old daughter they took away from me to the white man's land. She was only four when they took her and that was almost five years ago. I have not heard if she is alive or dead. Have you seen her? Is she well? Is she coming home soon?"

The missionary had no answer.

In Ottawa a man sat at his desk, puzzled. There was a pile of papers in front of him. Presently he picked up the phone and called another man and asked, "What are we going to do with these fifteen Eskimo children who are now well, and should be returned home? They can't speak a word of English; we don't know who they are or where they came from. These are the first to be ready to be returned, and there will be more to come yet. What are we going to do with them?"

3

Near Quebec City stands Parc Savard. This red-brick, square barracks-like building is a seamen's hospital that is possibly more drab inside than outside, where it resembles an austere prison. For years now it has been used as a treatment centre for Eskimos. Frequently down the steps and out into the street creep figures in night clothes and dressing gowns, voyaging into the unknown in an effort to go home.

Time after time, in spite of those who are brought back by the police, others attempt to escape, hoping they will be able to find their way back to their own country. Nothing could be as bad as the place where they live and where the attendants speak French; even the few Eskimos who speak English can't understand them. They realize only too well that once autumn settles in, there is no hope of their going home for at least another year, and in desperation they try to find their own way.

Bishop Marsh's letter produced considerable fallout, of course, though not precisely the result he might have preferred. The prime minister referred the matter to Jean Lesage, who was minister of NANR at the time. Lesage in turn referred it to his deputy minister, R.G. Robertson, to Paul Martin, the minister of Health and Welfare (H&W)

and to L.H. Nicholson, the commissioner of the RCMP. Memos flew in all directions. The commissioner of the RCMP was offended at the aspersions cast on his officers and, recalling Dr Moore's figures on deaths in mission versus southern hospitals, thought that the southern hospitalization program was best for the people even though it was difficult to implement and inevitably caused some hardship. Officials at NANR agreed with Bishop Marsh's objection to hospitalizing Inuit in isolation from their own people and supported the idea of constructing a few more small northern hospitals for bed-rest TB patients and others who did not require specialist treatment. H&W was firmly against this.

As a compromise, while still refusing to build more Arctic hospitals, Moore agreed to concentrate Inuit TB patients in groups of fifty or more in three or four sanatoria in the South and to have "substantial numbers of Eskimos" on the hospital staff. For its part, the Northern Administration and Lands (NA&L) branch, which was specifically responsible for Inuit administration, announced that it would appoint a social welfare person to cover the visiting of Inuit in hospital and the reporting to their families. But by March 1955, Lesage had decided that it would be wiser not to answer Bishop Marsh at all, beyond the acknowledgment already sent by the PM's office, because a reply would almost certainly revive the controversy.

Bishop Marsh, however, did not subside. He wrote again to the prime minister on 8 March, asking if any action had been taken regarding the matters raised in his previous letter or if he was mistaken in believing that the man the press called Uncle Louis was interested in the people of Canada. This resulted in a joint effort by the deputy ministers of NANR and H&W to produce letters to the prime minister from their respective ministers which would "fit together satisfactorily" and could to be sent on by the PM to Bishop Marsh. In due course this happened, and Bishop Marsh concluded from the PM's covering letter that he was satisfied with the present attitude and with the action being taken. As the bishop explained to Paul Martin, this left him free "to discuss or quote from this correspondence, or my article, to the press or to the public" without "embarrassing the government."

The bishop may not have achieved a reversal of H&W's policy of southern hospitalization, but his lengthy and fervent correspondence about the plight of Inuit patients (as well, probably, as the publicity and adverse reports about the 1954 Eastern Arctic Patrol) helped to force a greater degree of humanity into the system. In December 1955, as promised in March, NANR engaged a social worker, Walter

Rudnicki, to head a new Welfare Section of Arctic Division in the NA&L branch, consisting of himself, Leo Manning, and an Inuk interpreter, Paulette Anerodluk. And in the summer, Moore had begun the program to centralize the hospitalized Inuit. From the east, they were to go to the Mountain Sanatorium in Hamilton; from the central region, to Clearwater Lake or Brandon in Manitoba; from the west, to the Charles Camsell in Edmonton. While this did not always happen, it did mark a shift towards making it possible to develop more acceptable conditions for the patients. That year quite a few patients were transferred to the larger centres from hospitals such as St Boniface in Manitoba and Sacré Coeur in Cartierville.[34]

The 80 or so hospitals to which Inuit patients were sent in the period from the 1940s to the 1960s are listed in appendix 3. About 90 per cent of these patients were sent south because of tuberculosis.

The BCG vaccination program was slower to get underway. In their paper on tuberculosis among the Inuit, Grzybowski and his colleagues reported: "Immunization with BCG vaccine of infants and negative tuberculin reactors under the age of 25 started in the late 1940's; however, there was little uniformity in technique and coverage was small. Some BCG was given without prior tuberculin testing by the 'C.D. Howe' team and survey teams from Moose Factory in the James Bay and Northern Quebec regions."[35]

In 1952, Moore told the commissioner of the Northwest Territories that BCG had been used "fairly extensively in the more settled parts of the country" but that in 1951 it was given to only 275 patients in the territories.[36] A major difficulty in its use up north was that it could be procured in Canada only from either the University of Montreal or the Connaught Laboratories in Toronto and had to be used within ten days of manufacture. In 1954, however, Moore announced a "bigger and better BCG program." This probably applied mainly to his Indian clientele, since Grzybowski reports that, for the Inuit, the exclusive use of intradermal BCG vaccine began in 1965.[37]

In 1955 the IHS was renamed Indian and Northern Health Services (INHS) to reflect a new arrangement that extended its responsibility for health care to the entire population of the Yukon as well as the Northwest Territories (taken on in 1948). This was necessary because the local taxation base was too small to fund medical services for the increasing non-native population of the territories, and the INHS provided the services on a cost-sharing basis. Meanwhile, it continued to subsidize the small mission hospitals and to expand its chain of nursing stations in the Arctic. In 1947 stations were opened at Coppermine and Inukjuak, in 1949 at Kuujjuaq, in 1952 at Cape

Dorset and Lake Harbour, in 1955 at Iqaluit, in 1957 at Baker Lake and Hall Beach, in 1958 at Cambridge Bay, and in 1960–62 at Povungnituk, Salluit, and Kuujjuarapik.[38]

Such nursing stations still provide the primary level of medical care. They were designed for out-patient care and uncomplicated childbirth, and for emergency treatment or patients awaiting evacuation. They are equipped with examining rooms, basic diagnostic equipment including x-ray and some laboratory equipment, medical supplies and drugs, and a few cribs and beds. Their size and staffing depends on the size of the community. Originally there may have been only one nurse; today, there may be as many as half a dozen. In the Northwest Territories the nurses were almost always white, often brought in from outside Canada, and the rate of turnover was very high. The support staff was usually Inuit, consisting of a handyman, a clerk/interpreter, and maybe a community health representative, a nurse's aide, or a dental therapist.

Once the IHS campaign was well into its stride, the number of Inuit in the sanatoria climbed steadily, reaching a peak in the mid-1950s. Then both the numbers in the sanatoria and the death rate began to decline. Accurate and consistent statistics on the early incidence and mortality of TB among the Inuit, and on the number of Inuit having treatment, are almost impossible to find. As mentioned earlier, neither the IHS nor the Northern Administration branch at NANR had accurate records of who was in hospital or where until the later 1950s. The x-ray surveys covered only parts of the population, and even the census figures were incomplete because of the Inuit's seminomadic lifestyle and frequent inaccessibility. Add to this the changes in nomenclature and recording data as jurisdictions changed and as the different basis on which information about tuberculosis treatment was classified, and the picture becomes confused, to say the least. In addition, figures put out by the various departments involved in the administration of the North differ, and statistics within reports are clearly inaccurate in some cases.

In the 1950s, incidence could be estimated only from the x-ray surveys or from the number of patients admitted to hospital for treatment. In nine of the surveys carried out between 1950 and 1960, for instance, 38,709 x-rays were taken and 905 cases of new or reactivated TB were found, giving an estimated incidence of 2,338 per 100,000 population. The number of Inuit x-rayed in each of these surveys ranged from 585 to 9,512, and the incidence of TB ranged from 1.5 per cent to 8.5 per cent;[39] but smaller groups of children were screened in various school surveys.

Table 8
Inuit Tuberculosis Morbidity, 1953–62 (Rates per 100,000 Population)

| Year | Hospital admissions[1] | | | First admissions only (StatsCan.) | | New and reactivated cases | | |
	No.	Rate[2] Annual	4-year average	Rate Annual	5-year average	No.	Rate[2] Annual	5-year average
1953	376	3,961		–	–	–	–	
1954	420	4,424		–	–	–	–	
1955	950	10,007		–	–	–	–	
1956	870	9,165	6,889	–	–	–	–	
1957	583	6,141		–	–	194	2,044	
1958	547	5,762		2,292		231	2,433	
1959	490	5,162		1,913		125	1,317	
1960	448	4,719	5,448	1,845		156	1,643	
1961	566	4,782		1,560		120	1,014	1,690
1962	–	–		1,462	1,814	–	–	

Sources: Department of National Health and Welfare, IHS and INHS annual reports, 1954–61; Statistics Canada, tuberculosis statistics, morbidity and mortality, 1962, cat. 83–206; G.J. Wherrett, *Tuberculosis in Canada* (Ottawa: Royal Commission on Health Services, 1965).
[1] First admissions, readmissions, and transfers. Transfers equalled one-quarter of the total on average in the mid-1950s.
[2] Rates calculated by author, except for StatsCan. annual rates.

Until the 1970s, annual sanatoria occupancy figures were reported for the number of patients in hospital on 31 December each year; but as table 6 showed, these underestimate by about one-half the number of people treated in hospital each year. Many people were brought out for checking or through mistaken diagnosis (x-rays are not 100 per cent accurate as diagnostic tools, particularly when given under extremely difficult conditions). Some people were brought out, found not to be in need of prolonged hospital treatment, and discharged during the year, but most remained in hospital for more than a year, gradually increasing the size of the hospital population until the mid-1950s.[40] The average length of stay in hospital in the 1950s was 28 months.[41] Estimates of morbidity through the 1950s from various sources are given in table 8.

Mortality rates also could only be estimated, as Wherrett noted in his 1945 report, because of the very high proportion of deaths that lacked medical certification as to cause. Only in the case of patients dying in hospital or attended by a physician could a firm cause of death be given. Table 9, based on an analysis of death certificates,

Table 9
Inuit Tuberculosis Mortality by Certified Number of Deaths, 1950–60

	Canada					NWT	Quebec	Other[2]
		Origin not stated		All	Known	Known	Known	Known
Year	Total	No.	% total[1]	others	Inuit	Inuit	Inuit	Inuit
1950	3,670	254	7	3,377	39	26	13	0
1951	3,478	258	7	3,189	31	24	6	1
1952	2,536	188	7	2,294	54	39	15	0
1953	1,872	126	7	1,711	35	25	8	2
1954	1,630	147	9	1,463	20	18	2	0
1955	1,421	103	7	1,302	16	12	4	0
1956	1,281	112	9	1,147	22	22	0	0
1957	1,210	111	9	1,082	17	14	3	0
1958	1,055	91	9	952	12	9	3	0
1959	984	99	10	880	5	5	0	0
1960	828	82	10	738	8	7	1	0

Source: Statistics Canada, Canadian Centre for Health Information, Mortality Deaths (Tuberculosis) by Ethnic Origin, custom tabulation, 1992.
[1] Percentages calculated by author.
[2] Other provinces: Manitoba, one in 1953; Newfoundland, one in 1951 and one in 1953.

Table 10
Inuit Tuberculosis Mortality Rates, 1950–60 (Rates per 100,000 Population)

Year	According to Statistics Canada		According to Indian and Northern Health Service		According to Medical Services Branch	
	Annual	Average[1]	Annual	Average[1]	Annual	Average[1]
1950	411		–		718	
1951	327		–		476	
1952	569	435	–	–	588	594
1953	369		280		386	
1954	211		105		234	
1955	169		137		149	
1956	232	245	206	182	231	250
1957	179		134		167	
1958	126		58		155	
1959	53		46		79	
1960	84	111	45	71	76	119

Sources: Statistics Canada, Canadian Centre for Health Information, Mortality Deaths (Tuberculosis) by Ethnic Origin, custom tabulation, 1992; Department of National Health and Welfare, IHS and INHS annual reports, 1954–60 (excluding Labrador); and S. Grzybowski, K. Styblo, and E. Dorken, "Tuberculosis in Eskimos," Tubercle 57, no. 4, supp. (1976), from Medical Services Branch's data on Northwest Territories.
[1] Averages calculated by author.

Table 11
Population by Ethnic Origin (Inuit) Canada in Census Years 1951–81

Census year	Total population	Inuit	Inuit % of total population[1]
1951	14,009,429	9,493	0.07
1961	18,238,247	11,835	0.06
1971	21,568,310	17,550	0.08
1981	24,341,700	23,200	0.10

Source: Statistics Canada, Census of Canada.
[1] Percentages calculated by author.

gives the numbers of Inuit deaths known to have been from tuberculosis during this period. It must be regarded as a minimal estimate, because of the number of Inuit who died unattended by a doctor. Ethnic origin was reported on 90 to 93 per cent of certificates during this period, but some deaths where it was not recorded may also have been of Inuit patients. Estimated mortality rates through the 1950s from Statistics Canada and H&W are given in table 10. Inuit census population figures are given in table 11.

It had taken fifteen years, since the IHS launched its anti-TB campaign, for the organizers to get objective indications that the programs were being effective in controlling the epidemic, but by 1960 all the statistical indicators were becoming more positive – particularly the mortality rate. Dr Moore and his colleagues at headquarters probably felt vindicated by these results, despite the criticism and opposition which they had sometimes met. But the perceptions of those in the field, the implementers of the programs and the patients for whom all this effort was mounted, may have been rather different. The 80 per cent of the Inuit who lived in the Eastern Arctic were mainly served by the Eastern Arctic Patrol boat. A description of their experiences – and of those of the government workers on the boat – may help to flesh out the bare statistics.

CHAPTER SEVEN

The Eastern Arctic Patrol

"The ship was deep in misery. It was terrible because it was the ship which carried the Inuit away from their homes to the sanatoria in the south. And they were herded together in the foc'sle, in the hold of the ship in three-tiered bunks, mass-fed, mass-accommodated. In the stormy seas they were sick, they were terrified, they were demoralized. They were frightened of what was happening to them, of what was likely to happen to them."[1] This was Robert Williamson's recollection of the Eastern Arctic Patrol (EAP) ship, the *C.D. Howe*, on which he was a passenger in 1953–54. This vessel, specially designed for Arctic service, with a well-equipped medical section and separate quarters for the Inuit evacuees, was the main vehicle of the EAP from 1950 until the patrol was discontinued in 1969. For many hundreds of Inuit, it became almost synonymous with going out to hospital.

Through all the reorganizations and changes of policy that afflicted those charged with administering the North, the patrol made its annual voyage through the long, late Arctic summer days, ploughing through ice, storm, and fog, calling at tiny isolated settlements, supplying goods and personnel, carrying scientific expeditions, checking on administration and health, administering justice, dispensing medicine, and transporting Inuit to and from hospital and between settlements.

The main patrol was carried on the *C.D. Howe* or, until 1947, on the Hudson's Bay Company ship *Nascopie*, and left Montreal in July for Churchill, calling at various points on the way. After a week or so in Churchill, it left for the long trip round the Baffin and was back in Quebec City by early October, having called at 20 to 30 settlements in the three months and logged between 9,000 and 10,000 nautical miles (approximately 18,000 kilometres). A typical itinerary for the *Nascopie* was that for 1947 (see table 12). At most of the places she

Table 12
Nascopie's Itinerary, 1947

Nautical miles[1]	Port	Dates
–	Montreal (dep.)	5 July
1,040	Cartwright	10–11 July
740	Lake Harbour	16–19 July
200	Salluit	20–21 July
70	Ivujivik	22–23 July
120	Cape Dorset	24–26 July
260	Southampton Island	28–30 July
325	Akulivik	1–3 August
260	Inukjuak	5–8 August
500	Churchill	11–20 August
320	Chesterfield Inlet	22–25 August
370	Ivujivik	27–28 August
1,120	Clyde River	2–3 September
630	Fort Ross	7–8 September
290	Arctic Bay	10–11 September
110	Dundas Harbour	12–13 September
150	Pond Inlet	15–17 September
880	Pangnirtung	21–24 September
600	Lake Harbour	28–29 September
1,700	Montreal (arr.)	6 October

9,685 total

Source: National Archives of Canada, RG85, 78:201–1(22).
[1] One nautical mile equals approximately 1,852 metres.

called, the *Nascopie* was met by smaller ships, schooners or peter-heads, or even sled and dog teams, which took deliveries to the even smaller or less accessible posts. At Churchill she connected with a plane and with the train to Winnipeg.

There were always several smaller boats covering different parts of the Eastern Arctic waters. In 1947, for instance, besides the *Nascopie* and the government icebreaker *N.B. McLean*, which serviced the radio stations along with its ice-breaking duties, there were four other ships scheduled.[2] The *Fort Charles* operated from Moosonee on short trips covering the east coasts of James and Hudson bays as far north as Umiujaq and Sanikiluaq from June to September. The *J.H. Blackmore* sailed from Montreal in July to Ungava Bay and Hudson Strait settlements, returning mid-August. The *Neophyte* and *Fort Severn* operated out of Churchill through July and August, serving the west coast of Hudson Bay. The ships were always in a hurry and were subject to the unpredictable (and often violent) weather and ice conditions. Even on the itineraries, it was the exception rather than the rule to allow more than a day's stopover in a settlement. In all, besides Churchill and Moosonee, 40 settlements were included in the itineraries in 1947, most of them for only one visit in the season.

Until the end of World War II, the government generally paid the Hudson's Bay Company or the missions to transport its officials on their supply ships. The officials had, therefore, to submit to the conditions and priorities of the ships' owners which were, of course, to supply their posts and safeguard their personnel. For instance, the 1944 agreement between the Department of Mines and Resources (DMR) and the Hudson's Bay Company covering the use of the company boat for the EAP stated that the shipper, DMR, "will employ a duly qualified medical officer who shall complete the entire voyage at the expense of the Company and the said medical officer will, as required, during the currency of the said voyage give medical care and attention to the officers and employees of the Company and other passengers on board the said ship 'Nascopie' and all such services will be rendered free of expense to the Company"; and, further, that "the Company will, if required ... (c) permit the said medical officer to treat on board the said ship 'Nascopie' patients suffering from non-infectious disease; (d) supply suitable accommodation at Ports of Call to enable the said medical officer to treat patients ashore."[3]

When one considers the number of patients the doctor might need to examine and treat in a hurry, the infrequency of the visits, the preoccupation of the ship's crew and local HBC factor with off-loading supplies, and the fact that the predominant illness affecting the population – tuberculosis – is infectious, the difficulties must have seemed overwhelming. It is little wonder that Dr Ross Millar, the medical assistant to the deputy minister of health, wrote a plaintive letter to R.A. Gibson at DMR in November 1943 saying, "One of the outstanding points is that the doctor accompanying the 'Nascopie' has so little time or opportunity to question the Hudson's Bay Factor or examine patients, and I do not know how this situation can be helped. Probably in all the circumstances all that can be expected of the doctor is to do the best he can."[4]

After Health and Welfare became responsible for health services to the Inuit in 1945, the medical party was enlarged to include a dentist, an eye surgeon, and an x-ray technician, allowing better coverage of both diagnosis and treatment. But it was still of necessity a great rush, and a frankly production-line system was introduced. It was described in the *Beaver* as follows:

Soon after the *Nascopie* anchored, the Eskimos were brought on board in boat-loads and, under the guidance of Alex. Stevenson, assisted by Interpreter Sam Ford, they were put through the clinic in an orderly manner.

First came registration, sometimes both in Eskimo and English names, and of course, most important of all, with the official number given to each Eskimo by the Administration. Next came the chest X-rays. The Eskimos thought the "white medicine-man" strange indeed when, instead of facing the camera, they were asked to stand, stripped to the waist, with their backs to the lens. Then came the medical check-up and when this was finished the ocular team would take the patient in hand. Finally, if any dental trouble was discovered, the patients were passed on to Dr. Frank.

In this way a large number of Eskimos could be examined in a comparatively short time, though stormy weather and other delays in ship-to-shore communication would occasionally delay or disrupt the work of the medicos. All able-bodied Eskimo males were, of course, unloading the cargo scows as they arrived at the beach, and as this work goes on at most ports of call only at high tide, it meant that the workers had to be examined during the period of low-tides when they were not working. All was well organized, however, and the medical work went forward smoothly.[5]

The wreck of the *Nascopie* in 1947 temporarily interrupted this newly launched intensive medical survey approach, but with the maiden voyage of the *C.D. Howe* in 1950 it came into its own again.

The *C.D. Howe* was a coastguard ship operated by the Department of Transport (DoT). She was specially designed for the Arctic by German and Milne of Montreal, built in Quebec, and launched at Lévis in September 1949. A 3,660-tonne, 90-metre-long, ocean-going vessel, she was strengthened for use in ice, had a cruising range of 16,000 kilometres, and was capable of carrying 1,000 tonnes of cargo, 88 passengers, and a crew of 60 to 70. Besides passenger and crew quarters, there was a mail room, a hydrographic-charting office, a laundry, refrigeration space, and a small hospital. The latter included an operating room, a sick bay with beds for six patients, a dispensary, a complete dental office, an x-ray room, and a darkroom. The ship also had a helicopter and landing pad, and special attention had been paid to heating and to ventilation to eliminate condensation. There were separate quarters for the crew, for the first-class passengers, and for the Inuit, who occupied the forepart of the ship.[6]

On the *C.D. Howe*'s maiden voyage in 1950 the medical team included, besides the physician and the dentist, an x-ray technician and a medical attendant. Halfway through the voyage, at Churchill, the team was enlarged by a second doctor and a nurse from the

RCAF. In subsequent years the composition of the team varied slightly but always included a dentist and an x-ray technician. It also gradually increased in size. The number of passengers varied from year to year, depending partly on the ship's commitments to various government departments and partly on the number of Inuit returning from or going out to hospital. In 1950 there were 18 Inuit passengers as well as the government party. In 1951 the government party (consisting of patrol members, including the medical team, various radio technicians, RCMP officers, and others who were changing posts) numbered between 30 and 47 at different stages of the voyage; and there were 11 Inuit who were returning home. In 1953 there were 16 Inuit returning home but up to 68 in transit from one settlement to another because of "lack of game." In 1957 there were at one point 88 Inuit on board, but on average 50 in transit at a time.

The Eastern Arctic Patrol in the 1950s was the responsibility of the Arctic Division (at first of DRD, and after 1953 of NANR), which provided the officer in charge of the patrol. The actual work, however, required the combined efforts of at least five other departments – National Health and Welfare, Transport, Mines and Technical Surveys, the RCMP, and the post office – each of which had its own priorities. As can be imagined, there were strains between the various government officials. The 1951 sailing instructions from DoT to the skipper specified that the captain was fully responsible, that the senior DRD officer was in charge of all shore operations except cargo, and that everyone on board was under the captain's discipline.[7]

Instructions from DoT to Resources and Development stressed that passengers must comply absolutely with the master regarding times for boarding and leaving ship, and that DoT would not be responsible – even to loss of life – for passengers stranded at any point if they ignored his instructions about this. On boarding, the passengers had to sign a release of DoT responsibility for loss of property or life on the voyage, and no insurance was available. Passengers were warned to expect plain food, inconvenience, and hardship, and were required to be in good health.[8] In these instructions, the passengers referred to were of course the first-class passengers, members of the patrol, and sundry researchers, military police, meteorogical personnel, and so on – and not the Inuit evacuees.

Both H&W and DRD were concerned about the time allowed at ports for the medical and administrative parties to do their work, and they told DoT in 1951 that "it is essential that we have a minimum of 24 hours at each place and up to 48 hours at a few of the larger and more important centres."[9] But time remained short, and the clinic often went on into the early hours of the morning, sometimes even starting after 10 o'clock at night, in the effort to cover all the local population in the time allowed by the tides and before the ship had unloaded the stores and was due to sail.

The early years of the *C.D. Howe* patrol seem to have been very difficult and unpleasant even for the first-class passengers. Even in 1947, before the ship was launched and the *Nascopie* sunk, there had been anxiety about a switch from the experienced captain and crew of the HBC ship to a new vessel with an inexperienced captain, particularly in view of the incomplete charting of the hazardous waters.[10] In 1951 the DRD's officer in charge of the patrol complained in his report that the organization on board was not good and that the captain kept too much authority to himself, making the work of the patrol less efficient and unnecessarily uncomfortable. He gave the following examples: no sea biscuits were provided for Inuit passengers; no meal service was provided for first-class passengers after 6 P.M., though their working hours were of necessity very irregular because of the ship's sailing schedule (this meant that they had to prepare and wash up their own meals if they wanted anything between 6 P.M. and 7.30 A.M.); that meals in the captain's mess were good but the passengers' food was poor; that posts ahead were not informed of the ship's estimated time of arrival and consequently sick people could not be gathered together ahead of time. He suggested that more authority should be given to the officer in charge of the patrol.[11] This was done the following year, and the captain's instructions were modified to give the officer in charge of the EAP full responsibility for coordinating work ashore, or on board, of all departmental representatives except hydrographers.

Nevertheless, it took some time to get real improvements. In 1954, for instance, as mentioned in chapter 6, there was a spate of complaints. This was the first year that the Canadian government, rather than the United States, had done the sea resupply for the joint Arctic weather stations. The *C.D. Howe* was involved in this as mother ship at Resolute for two weeks, with the passengers transferring to the CGS *D'Iberville* late in the northern section of the voyage. B.G. Sivertz, chief of the Arctic Division, was officer-in-charge of the patrol for the first section, to Churchill, where he handed over to Alex Stevenson for the northern trip.

There were the usual medical and administrative parties on board; the civilian passengers included a geology professor from Carleton University and some journalists and CBC staff. Some of these people were shocked at conditions on the boat. Several passengers, at least one of whom was an ex-naval officer, wrote letters of complaint to Sivertz;[12] and Sivertz himself, who also was an ex-naval officer, put in a highly critical report, mainly on the ship's operation, which was duly handed on to the marine superintendent at the Department of Transport.[13] As well, the *Vancouver Sun* published an extremely critical article by Stanley Burke.[14]

Among the long list of complaints, many concerned the fact that safety and emergency procedures were inadequate and that some of the equipment was not in a condition ready for use. For example:

- Fire and lifeboat drills were rarely done (not even once in one five-week trip), and were carried out in a perfunctory and sloppy manner; the crew was not well trained in them.
- Fire hoses were not connected to the hydrants or nozzles, and hammers had to be used to free the hydrants from paint.
- Although there were three different and basically unilingual groups on board (French-speaking crew, English-speaking government officials and passengers, and Inuktitut-speaking Inuit) fire instructions were in English only, and thus neither crew nor Inuit could understand them.
- There were no instructions on boat drill for the Inuit and no emergency instructions in Inuktitut anywhere, despite the fact that most Inuit were on a ship for the first time and would not be likely to know what to do in an emergency.
- There were no visible provisions to get patients out of the sickbay to the lifeboats, and oil drums blocked the escape door (until Sivertz demanded their removal).
- There was no sea boat kept ready for launching, nor was there a trained crew in readiness. The only life-saving equipment in the barges (used to transport passengers) was four lifebelts.
- Oil drums were stowed around hand-steering gear, preventing its use.
- Watertight doors were unmarked, and there was no routine for closing them.
- Gasoline was stored under the helicopter platform, where it was very vulnerable to a helicopter fire.
- A case of dynamite was lying around for months (and even used as a seat on occasion) before it was safely stored.
- No-smoking regulations near gasoline were not enforced, and the crew often smoked near oil or gas drums.

Some complainants apparently felt that the crew generally consisted of inexperienced, unhelpful, and sloppy political appointees and that most government passengers took the patronage and inefficiency as a matter of course. Arising from this situation were the following criticisms:

- There was not one qualified deep-sea navigator on board, and the astronomical navigation procedures used "belong in sailing-ship days."
- There were only two deep-sea officers on board, and they were both in the engine room.
- The captain made no inspection rounds.
- Freight checking and handling was inefficient and haphazard, and crates were sent to the wrong ports – a serious matter in view of the fact that deliveries were made only once a year.
- The ship was very dirty, particularly the Inuit quarters and toilets, as well as the cargo barges that were commonly used to transport passengers.
- There were irregularities in the management of the ship's victuals and stores. For instance, different prices were charged in the canteen to passengers and crew; NANR was overcharged for the Inuit "lunch"; passengers and visitors were allowed to barter goods for the ship's supply of liquor; and the chief steward bought up crafts from the Inuit and sold them to the crew (who were not allowed to buy them directly from the Inuit) for racked-up prices.
- The ship's officers drank too much, and the crew were sometimes under the influence.

Other complaints concerned the restricted meal service (which had encouraged passengers to buy supplies and drink ashore at the settlements and to party in their cabins); the unavailability of insurance on personal property; and the "deplorable service given by the health authorities."[15]

Sivertz noted in his personal diary that some of the medical party drank heavily and were sometimes unwilling to carry on the survey at night when the ship's schedule demanded it.[16] He met considerable opposition when he suggested to the doctors that the *C.D. Howe* should be a "dry" ship or that drinks should be available only in the public rooms. He also noted in his diary that he considered the captain to be a competent man who probably lacked experience in sea-going ships that required discipline and routines in seamanship. Sivertz believed that the problems facing the captain might make it impossible for him to run an efficient ship, which Sivertz was sure the captain wished to do. As regards the state of the ship, the first mate told Sivertz that he was given only three weeks and nine men to prepare her after the winter lay-up, and Sivertz agreed that this was an impossibly short time. Sivertz felt some hostility from the ship's officers after his inspections of the EAP quarters and facilities, and because, as an experienced naval officer, he was constantly noticing the faulty maintenance and operation of the ship. But he thought that if he did not do something to improve matters, the ship would be in hazard. As he confessed to another passenger, he was terrified out of his life.[17]

In the crew's defence, it should be pointed out that, with the exception of the senior officers and engineers, they were for the most part a "green" crew every year, "recruited from the shores of the St Lawrence as a political patronage exercise." (This was before the days of the Public Service Employment Act of 1967.) They had little sea experience, though they sailed through possibly the most dangerous and difficult waters in the world, where help was far away and where water can kill in three or four minutes. They were inadequately trained, handicapped by the unilingual isolation of the groups, and probably fearful (with some justification) of catching TB from the Inuit passengers in the prow of the ship – though Betty Marwood, a social worker who went on later patrols, said that the Inuit quarters had to be put out of bounds to the crew because they were going down there to play with the children. Marwood noticed how very gentle the deckhands were with the children, particularly when helping them on or off the ship. "They handled those Inuit kids with love ... One chap, nicknamed Paul Bunion, was so gentle with them it was pure delight to see him; he just loved them."[18]

No major catastrophe seems to have occurred during the C.D. Howe's trips as a result of the deficiencies reported by Sivertz. As Williamson put it, "The ship managed to get itself around and didn't end up on a rock ... but that was probably as much luck as skill." But the lethargy and inexperience of the crew and the poor state of readiness of the equipment may well have been at least partly responsible for the death of one passenger. Stanley Burke's article reported that an Inuk boy, returning home after TB treatment, slipped off the Churchill docks and drowned. Burke said that although some of the crew could swim and the water in that area was not cold, the only action taken was to throw him a lifebelt, which did not reach him; and that it took more than twenty minutes to launch a boat.[19]

This spate of complaints, the publicity caused by Burke's *Vancouver Sun* article, and Bishop Marsh's "Cry the Beloved Eskimo" campaign all came around the same time and probably bore fruit. The following year, the medical staff had been changed, there was a new officer in charge of the patrol, and Sivertz was shortly to be promoted to a branch director. In 1956 an administrative assistant was added to the Northern Affairs team on the ship, and by then the new Welfare Section under Walter Rudnicki had been started at NANR. Rudnicki, who had already been alerted by Leo Manning about the problems of the Inuit patients, visited sanatoria across the country and was horrified at the lack of contact between the patients and their families.[20] Some children had been in the wards for six or seven years without any contact with their parents. Rudnicki recommended putting a welfare officer on the *C.D. Howe* to try to redress the situation. So in 1957 a social worker, Ruth Banffy, was for the first time included in the Northern Affairs team on the patrol to "prepare sick Eskimos for their evacuation to hospital and to make suitable plans for the families dependent on them,"[21] and Rudnicki went on the northern half of the voyage round the Baffin, as officer in charge of the patrol, to see the situation for himself.

Meanwhile, the annual surveys went on. The procedure through most of the 1950s was much as was described in the *Beaver* extract given earlier in this chapter. But that account does not tell the whole story. The medical party seems to have concentrated on efficient physical examinations, carried out in the minimum time possible, and on the physical separation of sick from well Inuit in order to give the sick the best possible physical treatment available at the time; but very little, if any, attention was paid to the effects of this separation on either the patients or their families, and there was little sensitivity shown in how it was done. From interviews with some ex-patients and with former government officials who were members of the patrol or passengers on the ship in the 1950s, the following picture emerges.[22]

The local administrator (usually the RCMP officer, HBC factor, or priest) was alerted if this was possible – for radio is not always reliable in the Arctic – of the ship's estimated arrival time and was expected to have arranged for all the Inuit to be on hand when the ship arrived. Sometimes a priest would connive at hiding people who were afraid they would be sent south, and sometimes Inuit in outlying camps would flee when they saw the ship coming or when they heard the helicopter, which was occasionally used to warn of its imminent arrival. When the ship arrived, all the Inuit in the settlement who were not busy unloading cargo were brought on board in the cargo barges, twenty or thirty at a time. Sometimes they came in their own boats. If the waters were very rough, they might be hoisted to the ship in a cargo sling. Once on board, they went through the screening system more or less in the manner described in the *Beaver* article.

Everyone's disc had to be shown and the number checked against government lists. This registration seems usually to have been the job of the official Inuit interpreter. Since the whole population was being seen, mothers came with small babies in their parkas, and dressing and undressing was difficult for them. The smell of sun-cured sealskin mukluks was sometimes overpowering in the crowded rooms of the clinic in the stern of the ship. Since everyone was under the pressure of time, and since there were few and often imperfect interpreters (a local person usually worked with the public health nurse, checking on immunization and so on), the Inuit were "shuffled through" mostly by signs. They had little chance of talking or arguing with the officials even if they felt so inclined. As they went through each stage of the screening process, a letter was marked on their palms to show that they had completed that stage. All the Inuit attending the clinic were served lunch on board: a mug of tea and a couple of hardtack biscuits.

When the doctors had made their final decision on whether an individual should go to hospital for treatment or stay in the North, the evacuees were sent down to the Inuit quarters in the prow of the ship and the rest were sent ashore. The evacuees were not allowed to go ashore to collect belongings, to say goodbye, or to make arrangements for their families or goods. If a mother was judged sick but her children were not infected, the children (sometimes including unweaned babies) were given to an Inuk woman going ashore. Fathers had no chance to arrange for someone to hunt for food for their families or to look after their dogs and equipment. Mothers had no chance to arrange for someone to care for their children or to sew and process the skins needed to keep the family warm. Virtually nothing was done from the social side. Those needing hospital treatment were kept on board, the rest sent ashore, and on sailed the ship to the next settlement.

Even on the rare occasions when an effort was made to explain to the family why it was essential for a family member to go out, and quickly, the partings were almost unbearable. Robert Williamson – who, as an Inuktitut-speaking passenger in the early 1950s, was roped in to help persuade a family from the Baffin to let their child go south – has been haunted for almost forty years by the desolation of the mother. She had already seen two of her children die at home from tuberculosis, and now had to sit by as Williamson carried her third sick baby off to the boat. Happily, this child recovered and now has children of her own.

On board, the Inuit shared a large room on a lower deck in the prow of the ship, with double- or triple-tiered bunks along the sides and with washrooms adjoining. Their menu was similar to that of the first-class passengers, though not always the same. It was sent from the galley in bulk containers, together with a pile of plates and cutlery, and served by the patients themselves. When there were a lot of Inuit on board, a still lower level had to be opened up. A total of 36 bunks was available in the two levels, but in 1958, when the ship brought out 83 patients, they had extra mattresses on the floor, stacked in the day, and two children to a bunk.

There was no segregation. They were all together – men and women, people from different settlements, children without their parents, mothers with young babies, and women looking after strange, lone children. They had no possessions but what they stood up in. They had no idea what was going on at home or what was about to happen to them, and no possibility of getting home without government help. They were unable to communicate with the crew or most of the government party and were now totally dependent on the authorities. And they were sick, unused to sea travel, confined for most of the time to the least comfortable and most crowded part of the ship, with little to do but worry.

Because communication was so poor between the hospitals and the settlements, and because so many of the patients taken out in the early days were far advanced in the disease and required many years of treatment (or indeed died of it in the South), the Inuit regarded going out on the boat virtually as a death sentence. This was particularly true of older people, who just wanted to die at home. Even if they knew there was a good chance that they would survive to return, they also knew that they would hear nothing of each other for years. It was little wonder they were upset. Robert Williamson felt their predicament keenly:

It was the coercive and insensitive way in which the people were picked up and herded into the ship and taken away. It was rather better for the patients who were being taken home from the south in the same ship. They were at least going home. But in many cases they had been traumatized by their experiences in the south and were apprehensive as to what they might find when they got home, what might have happened to their families. Sometimes they had no idea what had happened, they had had no communication; they had no idea where they were, or who had survived or who had given up on them, remarried or whatever.

And for the younger ones, children up to their early teens, who had been any length of time in the south, it was *terra incognita*. In their case, the hospital and the nurses had become home and the only people they knew, and going into the Arctic was going into the unknown. They may have been children going home, but they didn't know what home was like. Many of them were little southerners, with southern consumption needs and entertainment needs and language usages, with very little in common with the parents who yearned for them back home.[23]

Alex. Spalding, an interpreter on the ship from 1956 to 1959, when things were just beginning to improve, thought that the Inuit accommodation was reasonable and the food not too bad (the same as everyone else's, though not served so formally); and sometimes the Inuit could get their preferred game or seal meat brought on board when the boat called at a settlement. But the trips could be interminable. If the patients could not be sent south by train or plane from Churchill, they might be on the ship for two to three months – bored, sick, longing for the people they had left behind, and worried about their family's survival or their dogs and equipment that had been so summarily abandoned. Sometimes Spalding flew in the helicopter with the doctor to an outlying camp to try and persuade a family, or a sick member of the family, to come to the ship:

But they'd run away – they'd try to hide and not be there. It was always sad. It was disgusting, the whole thing was disgusting. We were just breaking into their lives for one, two, three, or four years. We didn't leave them any choice. A lot of times people who approached them weren't all that thoughtful; or if they were, they didn't have the means to really address their worries. People had a job to do and didn't have much time to do it. The white people on the boat hadn't lived there – they didn't understand the problems.[24]

(All the interpreters had lived in the Arctic, some for many years, and Spalding himself spent eight years with the Hudson's Bay Company in Repulse Bay before going to university and working summers as an interpreter for the patrol.)

This was the situation on board through most of the 1950s, though some action was taken to address the complaints raised in 1954. The 1957–58 sailing instructions, for example, differ in several respects from those of 1954. By 1957, the ship was designated as "dry." Only six cases of liquor, "for medicinal and rescue purposes only," were carried and these were under the complete control of the master. The Inuit visitors (that is, clinic patients) were provided with box lunches by NANR and with facilities for making tea in the Inuit quarters. The prices for canteen goods were specified and posted, and no financial arrangements were allowed to be made directly with the steward, who had to furnish accounts to DoT at the end of the voyage. And the arrangements for cargo manifests, accounting, and reporting generally were tightened up. The master and steward had to consult with the officer in charge of the patrol about accommodation on board; the officer in charge was responsible for informing the master how much time was required in each port to deal with patrol matters; and additional light refreshments were available from 10.00 to 10.30 P.M. each night. The members of the patrol, in their pre-boarding guidance paper, were reminded that "Eskimos are full Canadian citizens ... to be treated with the same dignity and under-standing as other fellow-passengers"; but that "the Eskimo quarters, in which tuberculosis patients may be found are out of bounds to all members of the Patrol, except with the permission of the O.i/c or the Senior M.O."[25]

As it happened, the patrol that year was even more difficult than usual.[26] At Churchill the ship picked up 76 patients returning home to settlements on its route between Churchill and Resolute Bay. It had discharged only 21 of these at Coral Harbour when a case of measles was confirmed among those returning and the whole group had to go into quarantine. No more returning patients could go home and no new patients could go to hospital, so the Inuit quarters were grossly overcrowded. Moreover, the ship was already committed to the Arctic resupply project at Resolute Bay, where it was needed to provide accommodation for the stevedores brought north on smaller ships. This arrangement was dependent on the freeing-up of the Inuit quarters. The ship's itinerary called for all returning patients to be delivered to their settlements before Resolute Bay and for any new patients picked up on the way to be flown south from Resolute.

Eventually, all the Inuit were put ashore at Resolute Bay and accom-modated in RCAF huts for treatment or vaccination. One doctor and two nurses from the ship accompanied them. While the ship was completing her resupply function at Resolute, the senior medical officer, Dr R.H.B. Sabean, wired the hospitals at which the returning patients had been treated to check which of them had a hospital record of measles. Those who did then continued home on the *C.D. Howe* at the close of the resupply project. The rest were kept in quarantine until they were deemed medically fit to continue their journey, either home or to hospital for TB treatment, whereupon they were flown out. The last 18 left for Grise Fiord, Arctic Bay, Pond Inlet, and Clyde River in a plane chartered by Health and Welfare in the early spring of 1958, having been at Resolute since the previous August.[27]

In her report on the 1957 patrol, Ruth Banffy recommended stream-lining the Welfare Section's operations with regard to the follow-up of patients, the administration of relief in the settlements, and arrangements on board for the Inuit. She also pointed out the need for improvement in matters under the control of the hospitals, notably the reports on patients and the inadequate clothing with which many patients were returning from hospital.[28] She then left the Welfare Section and was replaced on the patrol the next year by Betty Marwood.

Betty Marwood was disturbed by what she saw. She found it "a really shattering thing to see what was actually going on in my own country. You just don't treat people like that."[29] New to the job, she did not speak Inuktitut or know much about the North, so she just went along with the system for that year, doing what she could and thinking that she might leave at the end of the season and return to Children's Aid Society work down south. But near the end of the trip, at Iqaluit, she ran into a friend and "blew up in a rage," pouring out all the frustrations that she had had neither time nor opportunity to express on the ship. After she had calmed down, she decided to stay on and fight for improvements.

The Welfare Section was not trying to change the medical process. Betty Marwood, for one, is very proud of the unique Eastern Arctic medical patrol and the fully equipped hospital ship of Captain Fournier and his crew, which serviced, at great expense, the Eastern Arctic. She perceived the job of the social worker as being "to pick up from the medical people and deal with the social problems created by this system, by this having to take people out to hospital, to see that the families were cared for at the same time. It was a sort of assessment to see what needed to be done and then to do it."[30]

In 1960 the administrative function of the EAP was transferred to the new regional headquarters for Arctic administration at Iqaluit, and the importance of the ship's medical function increased accordingly. From then on, the senior medical officer from Health and Welfare was the officer in charge of the patrol, and the welfare officer was the senior Northern Affairs representative. In 1962, for instance, Dr Brian Brett was the officer in charge of the patrol, and the medical party consisted of five doctors (including a radiologist, an ophthalmologist, and an ENT specialist), five (or, for some stages of the voyage, six) nurses, two dentists, two dental technicians, and one x-ray technician.[31] Counting the social worker, translators, assistants, and ward aides, the medical party amounted to as many as 25 people in the 1960s. Betty Marwood was the welfare officer from 1958 to 1964, barring only one year. She had an administrative assistant and a translator working with her.

Despite the improvements, the patrols were inevitably stressful for the medical and welfare personnel. The ship still had to get round the settlements in the short season of open water and to contend with the unpredictable, sometimes violent weather. The broader range of health and social problems covered by the enlarged medical group meant that more work had to be crammed into the brief time available in each port. All the medical staff worked under pressure, and even with skilled interpreters, communication with their Inuit patients was very difficult for them, for Inuktitut had few medical terms. There were few opportunities for relaxation, sleeping was often disrupted by the ship's schedule and by the long hours of daylight, and accommodation was crowded. Colleagues in shared cabins often found that working, eating, sleeping, and socializing together for 24 hours a day was too much to endure. Eventually this was eased to some extent by cross-matching disciplines in the cabin allocation. Mealtimes were strictly kept. Patrol members were expected to "change for dinner," even when the clinic was running, and places at the captain's and chief engineer's tables were allocated according to seniority. But the 10 P.M. snack helped bridge the gap between the early dinnertime and breakfast, particularly on those occasions when the clinic operated through the late evening.

Betty Marwood was determined to improve conditions during her tenure on the patrol. She managed to persuade the H&W team and DoT to modify the survey procedure in three ways. First, since the welfare officer was the last "station" on the survey, she arranged that the doctor should tell her rather than the family which members, if any, had to go south, and that she should then tell the family. This, she found, lessened their anxiety, since she could immediately direct their attention to what to do about their family, their dogs, and so on, in their particular circumstances. Given a positive approach and the chance to discuss their situation, even through an interpreter, with a person trained to handle social crises, the patients or their relatives usually found solutions, suggesting suitable people to care for their children, hunt for the family, and cope with other tasks. If they could not find a solution themselves, the social worker helped; for example, by placing children, arranging supplementary food rations for the family, or arranging for transport to another community where there were relatives with whom they could live.

Second, Marwood obtained permission for the patients to go back on shore to make their arrangements, to collect things they wanted to take with them, and to say goodbye. The doctors had been fearful that they would not return, but Marwood found that no patients who said they would be ready for pick-up for return to the ship at a certain time ever let her down.

Thirdly, DoT agreed that the ship would defer departure until the social worker had completed her work in arranging for the care of the families, even if all the supply and medical functions had been completed well beforehand. This stemmed mainly from an incident at one of the DEW-line sites, staffed by an American unit, where an Inuk, employed by the site, lived with his mother and two much younger brothers. The mother had to go out to hospital, leaving nobody to care for the young boys, who then could not stay on the site. The family had relatives in a settlement farther north who could care for the children, so Marwood and the mother flew in the helicopter to the site to get a radio message to Iqaluit to arrange for a plane to pick up the boys and fly them north. Fifteen minutes after landing, when she had just found the superintendent of the site and had barely begun explaining the situation to him, the helicopter pilot called out to say that they had to leave: the ship had already sailed and he had only just enough fuel to catch it. Marwood had to choose between staying to ensure the care of the children (which would mean leaving the ship without a welfare officer) or abandoning the care of the children to the American officer. Fortunately, the American volunteered to see that the children were taken safely up north to their relatives, and he promised to care for them in the meantime; so Marwood and the mother flew back in the helicopter to the ship.

Marwood's reforms allowed more attention to be paid to alleviating some of the hardships and anxiety of the evacuees and their families, and helped to give the Inuit a little more control over their own affairs. The preferred solution to the problem of families deprived of provider or caregiver was for another adult in the family to take over the function. The second choice was for another adult in the community to take on the function, to foster the children or to hunt for the family. Only if these solutions were not possible would the family be broken up, with the children being fostered by relatives in another community or found foster homes by the social worker, who was by then established in Iqaluit. As a last resort, the children would be taken south with their mother and fostered there. In 1961, for instance, when 58 patients were flown south from various points along the ship's route, 28 children were placed in foster homes in the North; and along with the 47 patients who completed the voyage to Quebec City, there were six infants who were to be fostered down south near where their mothers were to be in hospital.[32]

As the patrol screened virtually all the communities every summer, it provided an opportunity to report back to the families on the progress of their relatives down south. This was the responsibility of the Northern Affairs welfare officer, and Marwood and the other welfare workers delivered any messages, tape recordings, or photographs sent up by patients in the sanatoria. A keen photographer herself, Marwood began to arrange for photos to be taken of the families in the North, which were later distributed to the relatives who were patients in the South. She also arranged for photographs to be taken of the new patients with their families before they left their settlement, so that they would have the pictures with them in hospital.

At first, Marwood commandeered passengers on the ship to act as photographers. To avoid mix-ups during the development process, both the photos and the person photographed were identified by a number. Marwood recalls that the first photographer "stuck their numbers on a label on their chest like a criminal! It was better than giving them the wrong picture, but it looked terrible."[33] She persuaded the department to provide a polaroid camera, and from then on, her assistant acted as photographer. Two pictures were taken of each family or patient and were developed instantly. One copy stayed with the family, the second was given to the patient.

Marwood's assistant was responsible for on-board recreation for the Inuit patients. The Welfare Section provided materials for making parkas, duffle socks, mitts, and knitted caps, as well as soapstone and tools for carving. Movies were shown in the Inuit quarters, and sessions of bingo and card games were arranged. Despite some risk of infection to themselves, the interpreters and welfare workers spent many hours with the patients. Clothes that would be more suitable than their own for the southern hospital setting to which the patients were bound – jeans, sweaters, dresses, pyjamas, and baby clothes – were provided, and toys for the children. So although the *C.D. Howe* remained "a rather sad vessel,"[34] the tedious and uncomfortable journey was made a little less onerous for the patients. It may even have helped to prepare them slightly for the totally unfamiliar life that awaited them in hospital.

CHAPTER EIGHT

Life in the San.

There were many routes to the sanatoria, most requiring a stopover, sometimes for a week or more, before transport was available or the weather was right or the group big enough to move south conveniently. The Inuit left the Arctic by ship or plane and usually transferred to another plane or to a train for their journey farther south. Some arrived in small groups or singly, but most arrived in large groups following the spring or summer x-ray surveys. Post-survey arrivals at the two principal centres where Inuit were treated, the Charles Camsell Indian Hospital in Edmonton and the Mountain Sanatorium in Hamilton, required special arrangements by the hospitals, which were notified in advance about each flight bringing in patients from the North.

The wardmaster in charge of orderlies at the Camsell hospital went to the airport with transport to meet the planes, which arrived in the evening and carried 24 to 30 patients at a time. Often the patients were still dressed in their furs – suitable for the High Arctic but very hot clothing for Edmonton. Sometimes a mother arrived carrying a baby in the hood of her parka, the baby wearing nothing but a tuque. The hospital set up a reception centre in the big recreation hall and handled the admissions in "something of an army-style fashion," according to Elva Taylor, director of nursing at the Camsell from 1947 to 1971.[1] Besides the admitting doctors and nurses, the reception team included an interpreter if possible. The first concern always was to provide a good meal for the patients. Hot soup, beef stew, raw frozen fish, and lots of tea were always popular. After the meal, the regular admissions procedure was followed: the patients were examined, whatever information had come with them was checked and recorded, and they were assigned to wards. As far as possible, the hospital staff put people who had come from the same area together in the same room; if there were only a few Inuit in a ward full of Indian patients (who were in the majority in the hospital), they would put the Inuit in beds side by side or opposite each other for company and communication.

Communication was always a big problem, since few of the Inuit spoke English and none of the staff spoke Inuktitut. The differences between Inuktitut dialects added to the confusion; the patients who could speak some English and tried to interpret often found they could not understand patients from another district. So explanations and instructions had to be by signs. After a while, more patients learned enough English to be able to help translate, but initial adjustment to the hospital setting and routine was always made more difficult by the language problem.

The patients were taken to the wards by wheelchair or stretcher and, if well enough, given tub baths – a totally new experience for 99 per cent of them. Then they were dressed in hospital clothing (their furs placed in storage) and put to bed, which was also a foreign experience for the majority, who were accustomed to a sleeping platform at one side of a snow house. One former nurse remembers having problems with an elderly Inuk woman who repeatedly got out of bed and went to sleep on the floor. In retrospect, the nurse thought that the patient probably felt very insecure lying on something so high off the ground, but patients' letters suggest that she probably disliked the soft mattress and preferred the hardness of the floor.[2]

Everything was strange to the Inuit: the big solid buildings, the beds, the bathrooms, the flush toilets, the basins with running water, the heat, the food, the language, the clothes, the activities – or lack of them – and the bed rest that was expected of them. But the staff found that the Inuit patients were generally very observant and were good at understanding signs, and so long as they realized that something was important for them, they cooperated very well.

Similar procedures went on at the Mountain Sanatorium in Hamilton when patients were flown there from the Eastern Arctic. Mini Aodla, a teenage patient who later became an official interpreter with the Welfare Division, helped interpret for the first planeload of Inuit patients to travel directly from Iqaluit to Hamilton, in 1953. One of the few patients who could speak English, she went with the head nurse to meet the plane at about three o'clock in the afternoon of a very hot day in one of the hottest summers that Hamiltonians remembered. The Inuit had been in the plane for many hours and were wearing their sun-cured caribou-skin parkas and outfits. Many of the mothers had infants in the backs of their parkas, with diapers of

Arctic moss or an extra piece of fur, and the heat and smell in the airplane was terrible.

Mini Aodla found it all very sad: "The thing that hit me the most was how the women talked, some of them saying, 'Where have we gone to? Where are we? Look at all this cement. There's no land here. Where are we going to be put, and what else are we going to ride in? That must be where we are going to' (looking at the airport building). All these questions were just going in their heads, talking to themselves, some of them talking to each other, you know."[3] None of the group spoke English. Mini Aodla was asked by the nurse to tell them to gather their stuff and get into the big van or ambulance for the drive to the hospital. When she spoke to them in Inuktitut they were surprised, and she was very insulted because they had "totally thought I was a white woman."

The patients were taken to the main building at the sanatorium for registration. The process took hours, partly because of the confusion over names and numbers. Since the Inuit did not use surnames at that time, the admitting officers often did not realize that wives, husbands, and children were members of the same family. The southerners had difficulty spelling the unfamiliar names, and as this was before the era of social insurance numbers, they were unaccustomed to identifying people by numbers. Mini Aodla felt caught between two cultures, trying – with only partial success – to explain each to the other. It took about a month, she recalled, before they had all the names straight and correctly spelled.

Allocating patients to wards and getting them there was also time-consuming. The group consisted of people with different degrees of infection and included men and women, teenagers, young children, and babies, some of whom were well and were simply accompanying their mothers. These groups were normally treated in different wards, often in different buildings spread throughout the hospital grounds. Mini Aodla described how upsetting this was for the patients: "Women were crying, really, because they were being separated from the children and the babies they had at their breast. They were saying, 'Where is it? Where is it going to be put? Will I see the baby now and then?' It wasn't because the hospital workers were mean or anything, it was for health reasons that they were separated. The Inuit patients couldn't understand that, they couldn't see that at all."[4]

The natural confusion of the patients in these totally unfamiliar surroundings is reflected in the account of Sarah Saimaiyuk, who went out in the early 1950s.

We used to live in a camp near Pangnirtung. We were told that we had tuberculosis, and we were brought to Pangnirtung. We stayed at the hospital there, waiting for the airplane to take us down south. When it arrived, it landed on the water and anchored quite a distance from shore.

We were taken to the airplane by boat and having never seen an airplane before, I was very puzzled. "I wonder where the entrance is?" I thought. "The only thing that looks like a door is underwater! How are we going to get inside? How does it fly? We might sink if it's unable to fly!"

During the flight we got very thirsty, and we were frightened. My little sister, who was only a baby then, started crying. I was so thirsty that my mouth got very dry, and we couldn't tell the qallunaat [white people] who were with us, because we didn't speak their language. Although I knew the word for water in English, I didn't say anything, thinking there was no water in the airplane. I was so frightened of the qallunaat.

Finally we landed, and I overheard somebody saying that we were now in Moose Factory and not too far away from Hamilton. We were taken to a residence for patients. When we got there, there seemed to be no one in the building, but when I looked out through the window I saw one man standing outside.

I was dying for a smoke. Thinking they may not allow it, like in the Pangnirtung hospital, I didn't even try. I was too scared to ask.

In the residence I saw a wooden bed that had been used by a patient coming back from Hamilton. On it he had written the names of all the patients, and messages. That's how I learned that I was going to Hamilton. I think he must have learned to speak English because some words were in English.

We were then taken to a train and as we started to go, I noticed the air felt very stuffy. I felt like I was going to suffocate! When I looked up, all I could see were lights. Later, I learned that we were going underground. My little sister must have been taken by a nurse and was in another section. My little brother was with me. We travelled all night long, but this time it was more comfortable than in the airplane. We could drink water whenever we got thirsty and there was even a washroom! It seemed like we were in a house. There were a lot of Inuit patients on the train.

When we were told that we had arrived in Hamilton, I was just over-whelmed. "So this is where qallunaat come from," I thought. All the children were taken to one hospital, probably a children's hospital, and we adults were taken to another. When they took my little sister Lucy away, I cried because I wanted her to be with me. When I got to the hospital, all my clothes were taken away from me, maybe because I was more infected than the others. I never thought I was that sick.

All this time there were no interpreters. In the hospital I met Inuit from Povungnituk for the first time. I found out they could understand and speak English. I was then given a jar. An Inuk from Povungnituk tried to explain to me what to do with it, but I couldn't understand her because her dialect was so different from mine. Since I couldn't understand her, she just ran to her room in embarrassment. This made me feel terrible, as I began to believe I would never be able to communicate with them. Later on I found out the jar was for spitting.[5]

Titus Allooloo remembers coming out as a six-year-old in the early 1960s, when he sailed to Quebec City on the *C.D. Howe* and then went on to Hamilton by train. Allooloo spent about two months on the ship, on the second level down in the forepart:

It was foreign to me. The people were foreign to me, I couldn't speak the language, I didn't have the right clothing – I only had sealskin kamiks and parka. And the crew on the ship – some of them were quite good; they used to give me ten cents so I could buy a pop or something. The money was foreign to me, too, and the food ... The first two weeks, I think, I was basically sick, motion sickness. I couldn't eat, I couldn't do anything. I was sick, throwing up all the time. Then after that I was ok. I didn't get sick any more. It was quite a different experience!

Most of the ship's crew were fine. Some were not so nice. The ship's crew were mostly French. The nurses and others, doctors, were mostly English-speaking people ... There were nurses that regularly came around to check with us. At certain times I could go on deck. But there were some restrictions. When we were going through Labrador Sea it got really, really rough, and then we were basically confined to the inside of the ship. We couldn't go to the main area of the ship, towards the back [where the canteen was], so somebody had to go over there for us; these were mainly interpreters on the ship – I forget their names. Sometimes they were nice, sometimes they were not so nice.

We went to Quebec City. I remember going onto the docks, seeing whole bunches of people. That was amazing to me, the number of people that came to see us. Also big buildings, trees, roads, and cars. It was amazing. And I think we went out – I can't remember how we got off the ship – I think we were into the car. And then the next thing I remember was going on the train. That took a couple of days, I think, or overnight. I kept remembering seeing the cattle on the fields. That was amazing to me, and the horses, and the green fields. Then we got into Hamilton, we got into the car, and then we were checked into the hospital.[6]

Almost invariably, the first routine in the sanatorium was full bed rest. As Elva Taylor said, "Rest, rest, rest, and rest, as that was mainly the treatment we had, that and surgical procedures." The patients were at first allowed to do very little for themselves, but their activity was increased if their regular x-rays showed improvement. The Camsell activity routines in 1948, for instance, were:

Routine 1 – Complete bed rest. Complete bed bath. Mode of transportation, e.g., stretcher or wheelchair to be designated by ward doctor.
Routine 2 – Patients up once a day 11:00–11:15 a.m. (15 minutes only). Not to get up to have bed made. Routine twos may wash their hands and face only. Complete bed rest.
Routine 3 – Patients up twice a day for 15 minutes in a.m. when beds are being made, and from 3:15–3:30 p.m. Routine threes may wash face, hands and arms.
Routine 4 – Patients up to bathroom when necessary. NOT up after 4:00 p.m. May bathe all but their legs and back.
Routine 5 – Allowed up on the ward except during rest periods. May take a tub bath once a week. May do own shampoos. On wing wards down to meals at table. May walk to X-ray, lab and dentists.
Routine 6 – Allowed up except during rest periods. Tub baths (may do own shampoos). Exercise off ward between 11:00 a.m. and 4:30 p.m. except during rest period: 1) to Canteen, 2) walking in park area in front of hospital ONLY.
Church – Routine four people go to church once a month. Routine five and six people go to church every Sunday.
Visiting – Friday 3:30–4:40 p.m. is visiting time. Routine six people only, may visit patients in the hospital, with written permission from the ward doctor. All other patients may have visiting arranged by application.
NOTE: No patient is up before 8:00 a.m., regardless of routine.[7]

All types of tuberculosis were found among the Inuit patients: primary to far advanced, pulmonary, bones and joints, meningitis, renal, lymphatic, miliary. When the IHS mounted its attack in earnest on the disease in the late 1940s, there were no drugs available for the treatment of the disease. Dr William Barclay, one of the doctors at the Camsell, has described the treatment possibilities:

Bed rest, surgical collapse of the lung, and fixation of joints by plaster made up our therapeutic armamentarium. We employed these treatments more on blind faith and trust than on any scientific evidence that they were effective. Rest was the cornerstone of therapy and it was rigorously enforced through six routines of activity. Routine "1" was total bed rest and the patient barely moved, even to feed himself. Routines were changed as Meltzer[8] judged the disease to be improving or worsening, and the patients' hopes rose and fell as they either moved up or down the activity scale. With no television, few radios and many of the patients unable to read and hospitalized far away from home and friends, it was a cruel existence.

Surgical treatments, performed under local anesthesia, consisted of: thoracoplasty, pneumothorax, pneumoperitoneum and phrenic nerve crush.[9] Thoracoplasty was a painful and deforming procedure and, although Herb was highly skilled in the use of local anesthesia, only Matt's kind and gentle manner, as he sat by the patient's head, made the procedure tolerable. Pneumothorax fills were given twice a week to as many as fifty patients at a session. Herb fluoroscoped the patients and Matt, Margaret and I did the treatments with Miss Hall running the whole show with production line efficiency.

We had so many orthopedic cases that Margaret and I spent most of our afternoons applying plaster casts. It was not entirely a pleasant task since the old casts that we first had to remove were often filled with stench of suppurating fistulae. The children resented being immobilized and did their best to prevent us from applying a cast from which they couldn't subsequently wiggle free.

The most heartbreaking chore was intrathecal streptomycin rounds. When first made available [1944], streptomycin was scarce and expensive, and we had no clear direction as how best to use it. Since tuberculosis meningitis was uniformly a fatal disease, we used our scarce new drug for its treatment. We gave the drug both intrathecally as well as intramuscularly, and Margaret and I made regular rounds to inject the drug through a spinal tap to the children who dreaded the whole procedure. Since the tubercle bacillus developed resistance to the drug, we saved very few of those early cases. Not until we had a second drug, PAS, did meningitis yield to treatment.

Many of the children suffered from scrofula, tuberculosis affecting the skin over the neck, and under which were tuberculous lymph nodes. We soon learned that tuberculosis could affect every part of the body. Every joint in the body: hip, knee, ankle, wrist, spine, shoulder; none were immune. Kidney, bowel, brain, breast, eye, skin: wherever you looked you could eventually find it. A specialist in the field of TB had to be a generalist in so far as medicine was concerned.[10]

These treatments, together with Isoniazid (INH) which came into use in 1952, remained the main arsenal of the sanatoria through the 1960s until Ethambutol (EMB) and Rifampin (RFN) were introduced in 1969–70. The drugs allowed less dependence on bed rest and surgery, but in the 1940s and 1950s these were extremely important.[11]

Many of the patients did not feel particularly sick, hated being in bed all the time, and did not understand that it was essential. The staff sometimes resorted to physical restraint to keep them at rest. Methods of restraint included harnessing patients to the bed or putting a plaster cast on both legs. Titus Allooloo recalls that when he was caught with his harness off he was given a strapping. An article in the *Camsell Arrow* of December 1947 mentions an outbreak of "Castitis," which "is caused directly from Cantstayinbeditis."[12]

The hospital staff were generally very conscious of the need to keep their patients occupied and interested in living, but in the early years, particularly where there were only a few Inuit patients, they were handicapped by communication difficulties and lack of resources. Patients from the South could not only communicate easily with the staff, they could read the magazines and books available, listen to radio plays or talks, and most had money to buy comforts or materials to help keep themselves occupied. The Inuit patients usually had their Inuktitut Bible or prayer book with them and little else. Few had any money, and everything around them was available only in a foreign language.

The Northern Administration and Lands (NA&L) branch of the Department of Northern Affairs and National Resources, which from 1951 to 1959 was responsible for Inuit affairs apart from health, was slow to take action. The Indian Affairs branch, which at that time was under the Department of Citizenship and Immigration, provided teachers for the large number of Indian patients in hospital, and when Inuit were in a sanatorium that also served Indian patients, the teachers sometimes tried to accommodate them too. But as the Inuit came south in increasing numbers, this became more difficult. Not only were the teachers overloaded, but language was a barrier and the educational background of the two groups was usually very different. So eventually Indian Affairs refused to include the Inuit in its classes unless NA&L engaged – and paid for – additional teachers to cover the extra work.[13]

For instance, in 1952 there were 88 Inuit patients at Parc Savard in Quebec City who had no academic or handicrafts teacher. In the spring, James and Alma Houston of the Canadian Handicrafts Guild in Montreal gave two weeks' instruction there in carving, knitting, and elementary subjects, but by July the Houstons had moved to Cape Dorset, and J.G. Wright of Arctic Division was writing to the acting director of NA&L that "we may be open to serious criticism if we fail to seize the opportunity to provide some elementary education to the large number of Eskimos in the Hospital."[14] Unfortunately, NA&L had made no provision in its estimates for this and had to scramble to find money until the next fiscal year. Nevertheless, things had improved a bit by November. When Leo Manning visited the hospital that month, he reported that 12 Inuit children were attending the hospital school and were doing well, and that an extra teacher had been engaged for them and would start work in mid-November. In May 1954, NA&L engaged a handicraft instructor, Harold Pfeiffer, for Parc Savard, and a loud speaker system was installed in the wards to help expand the instruction possibilities.

At the Charles Camsell Hospital, Indian Affairs teachers had been running a school since 1947, and in May 1953 NA&L began to pay for an extra teacher to cover its responsibilities to the Inuit. This school covered Grades 1 to 10, plus some commercial subjects, and all teaching was done on the wards on a one-to-one basis. The hours were 11.00–12.30 A.M. and 3.15–5.00 P.M. Both adults and children, when well enough, were included in the classes. For the children, the aim was to start or to continue elementary school education, as appropriate. For the adults, the aim was twofold: to increase their skill in reading English, and to develop skills that would lead to employment within the scope of whatever physical disabilities the patients might be left with on leaving hospital. All the classes were taught in English.[15]

This was the pattern at most of the sanatoria, including the Mountain Sanatorium in Hamilton, where activities for southern patients had been well organized since the 1920s. The first sanatorium in the world to provide earphones for each bed (1922), it had a telephone line from McMaster University to carry courses of lectures on various subjects.[16] In 1943 the CBC had helped the hospital adapt its radio programs to make them more appealing to patients, and by 1951 the hospital had a flourishing school with seven teachers. At the height of the southern hospitalization program in the 1950s, the hospital's education department under George Young had up to 30 full-time teachers working on much the same system as at the Camsell.[17] It also had a few part-time teachers, some of them Inuit patients teaching Inuktitut to the children. In 1955 one of the NA&L teachers, Raymond Gagné, arranged for an outline of essential information for newly admitted Inuit patients to be taped in Inuktitut by Leo Manning.[18] As well, groups of patients were taken to the laboratory to see a culture of TB bacilli under a microscope so that they could better understand the nature of their disease. Gagné later learned Inuktitut, introduced an Inuktitut primer for Inuit children at the sanatorium, and held classes in Inuktitut for the staff.

As some of the young people stayed several years in the sanatoria and were generally enthusiastic learners, there were quite a few success stories among the graduates from these schools. In December 1953 the Camsell school principal reported, "An Eskimo lad who has been in hospital for four years and who has had a thoracoplasty and is a double amputee, has just finished four months of training in handling tools. He is now ready for training-on-the-job in cabinet making. Another Eskimo lad, an ex-patient, is to attend university this fall to train as a teacher."[19] In July 1955 a young Inuk woman, who had come south as a girl with her mother, first to Moose Factory and then to the Mountain Sanatorium, graduated from Grade 8 and was accepted into the nursing assistant course at Hamilton General Hospital.[20]

The main occupational activities of the adults were carving for the men and sewing for the women. Soapstone carving was sometimes frowned upon because it created a fine dust that was bad for the lungs, and the carvers had to wear masks. But it was the preferred medium, and by 1958 the patients at the Mountain Sanatorium were turning out about 200 carvings a month at a retail value of more than $10,000 a year.[21] The sanatorium ordered regular shipments of soapstone from a Quebec quarry and peddled the carvings for a 30 per cent commission. At Parc Savard the carvers were paid in cash or tobacco, while at the Camsell all patients were paid monthly a nominal amount of cash for their work.[22] The women made mukluks, mitts, even parkas, from furs and materials donated to the hospitals. They became very skilled with sewing machines. At the Mountain Sanatorium they made most of the pyjamas and nightgowns, clothing that the hospital had formerly bought. They were paid in lengths of material, with which they made clothes for themselves or their families. At the Camsell in the 1960s, when the occupational therapy department was allocated more space in the redesign of the hospital, weekly cooking sessions were organized for the women patients.

Dances, entertainments, movies, Christmas celebrations, and, at the Camsell, a summer picnic were arranged for the patients, and some local service organizations helped supply radios and gifts for them. One primary class at Hillfield School in Hamilton regularly "adopted" four Inuit children at the Mountain Sanatorium and sent them fruit at Thanksgiving and gifts at Christmas.[23] The patients themselves put on group entertainments and gave talks over the hospital radio. In 1954, after a visit to Parc Savard, Leo Manning reported that two violins that had been sent to two of the patients "were very much appreciated and have helped to provide a lot of good entertainment for the Eskimos. A tape-recording of songs, square dances, violin and accordion solos was made by the Eskimos and some of the Indians and it is very good. Mr. Lariviere is sending the recording to the Educational branch."[24]

Church services were held at the hospitals and often relayed to the wards, where the patients could follow them through their headphones; the Inuit patients often followed both the Anglican and Roman Catholic services. Missionaries from the North came regularly to the hospitals, carrying messages to and from relatives in the settlements. Leo Manning and, later, workers from the Welfare Division also visited the hospitals and collected tape recordings and photographs from patients to include on the summer surveys and patrols or on the Christmas mail airdrop, which was carried out round the settlements by the RCAF. The Camsell hospital arranged with CBC Winnipeg in 1955 (and later with CBC Inuvik) to play tapes from patients on their "Northern Messenger" program. In the 1960s, tapes were also made by relatives in the settlements and sent south for the patients in hospital, sometimes being relayed to the whole group in the hospital auditorium.

For patients who were well enough and no longer infectious, visits within the hospital were allowed, and trips outside were organized to shopping centres and factories. Some hospital staff invited patients to their homes. Many patients were fascinated with the domestic and farm animals they saw on trips outside the hospital, for they were totally unfamiliar with cows, horses, cats, and tame dogs. If the sanatorium was in a town or village, such as Weston or Ste-Agathe, the patients could go downtown to shop or for walks. At Ste-Agathe, which took a large number of Inuit patients in the 1960s when the sanatorium at Moosonee closed down, this occasionally led to a patient returning from an outing somewhat the worse for drink. At Hamilton's Mountain Sanatorium, which was less conveniently placed for shops, some of the young men found that they could snare rabbits in the grounds, and they cooked the meat on the ward hot-plates.

At the Camsell hospital great efforts were made to give the patients food that they liked, including frozen raw fish and wild meat such as venison or buffalo, when available. But generally the patients had to adapt to the hospital diet considered good for tuberculous patients. New arrivals would often eat only the meat or fish and leave the salads or vegetables, which they considered mere grass, not real food. The food was one of the aspects of life in hospital that was most disliked by the patients, though some of the children, hating it at first, later came to love it and missed it when they returned north.[25] The Inuit also found the heat and the soft beds very oppressive, in both the un-air-conditioned summers and the centrally heated winters.[26] At the Camsell hospital, they were really comfortable only in the winter rest periods, when they had the windows open and the ward temperature was just high enough to keep the radiators from freezing.

The closeness of the patients in hospital and their longing for their own country and the families so far away were particularly noticeable at Ste-Agathe. At all the hospitals, when patients were leaving to go home, they visited the other patients from their district to collect messages and perhaps gifts to take back to the relatives. But at Ste-Agathe all the Inuit patients fit enough to do so used to get up to see the lucky person off, even though the transport to Montreal airport left soon after 4 A.M. to catch the 6.30 A.M. flight to Iqaluit.[27]

Sometimes their unhappiness led them to disaster. David Mike-yook, a 60-year-old man from Kuujjuarapik, was one of a handful of Inuit in the Mountain Sanatorium in Hamilton in 1952 (the December 1952 nominal roll showed four patients there). Mikeyook had arrived at the sanatorium from Moose Factory in February of that year and was very anxious to go home by Christmas. But in September the doctors told him that although he was well enough to have limited walking privileges, he was not yet well enough to leave. On 1 October he walked out of the hospital, wearing pyjamas, light summer pants, and a dressing-gown; he had a jackknife and some razor blades with him. Despite a search and despite police, radio, and newspaper appeals giving his description, Mikeyook was not found until 29 November, when a 12-year-old boy came upon his body in a ravine about a kilometre from the hospital. Mikeyook had died only a few days earlier from starvation and exposure.[28] It is not known what was in his mind – whether he was trying to get home, whether he thought he could live outside the hospital, or whether he simply could not stand being inside any longer. It seems unlikely that he simply wished to die, since he had supported himself for two months in the brush on the hillside near the hospital, possibly using his hunting skills and snaring rabbits. One must wonder how thorough the search could have been, considering that Mikeyook was sick and lacked the wherewithal to get very far. The RCMP informed his next-of-kin through the Inukjuak police detachment, and Resources and Development paid for his burial in a pauper's grave in Woodland, the Hamilton municipal cemetery, on 3 December. Other Inuit tried a different form of escape: there are said to have been several cases where patients either tried to commit suicide or succeeded in it.[29]

Despite the efforts of some sanatoria staff to help the patients understand the nature of their disease and the reasons for certain treatments, there were many misunderstandings. Joanasie Salomonie, who came out on the *C.D. Howe* in 1954 and spent two years in Parc Savard, Quebec, thought that the doctors were experimenting on them – "a medicine experiment using different things on us," he said. "I'm sure they were practising on us because there were so many patients there."[30] In a sense he was right, of course: the doctors were not sure about the correct dosages or best applications of the new drugs just coming in, but were probably eager to use anything that offered an improvement over the treatments previously available for tuberculosis. Later, in 1959, Salomonie went to the Mountain Sana-torium where, he said, "there was a different treatment again. At that time, I guess, it was almost the right kind of medicine then."[31]

Another patient at the Mountain Sanatorium – an Inuk who spoke no English – was treated by a Chinese doctor. He assumed that the doctor was a fellow Inuk, but the doctor did not speak Inuktitut to him – simply came each day, smiling, even laughing, and said a few unintelligible words in English. The patient struggled to work out why a fellow Inuk would behave in this manner. The only explanation he could come up with was that there must be some sinister intent – that he was going to die and that was why he had been brought there. Later, when he understood English, he realized his mistake, but his first weeks in the sanatorium were made much more frightening by this misunderstanding between himself and the well-intentioned doctor.[32]

Most patients, particularly the older ones, undoubtedly were homesick and lonely. Dr Todosijczuk recalls the Inuit and northern Indian patients at Ste-Agathe sitting completely alone on a Sunday visiting day while cars streamed up with visitors for the rest of the patients, who came mostly from Montreal. But however unhappy and lost the Inuit may have felt, most of them appreciated the care and concern of the doctors and nurses, were very good patients, and seemed grateful for being cured. As Mini Aodla said, "It was terrible, but it was a war. The people were dying. They had to do something."[33] On the whole, the Inuit thought they were treated very well in hospital, even though they did not enjoy the experience, and many were glad of the educational opportunities they had and the new friends they met there. Yet while adults and teenagers could take advantage of the opportunities offered, they did not forget their language or the skills needed to live in the North. As one patient from Ste-Agathe put it after a visit to Montreal, "Well, it's magnificent, it's everything. But, you know, *I* can live in Montreal and I'll survive. But if a Montrealer is to go up north, *he* will not survive."[34]

CHAPTER NINE

After the Hospital:

Going Home, or
a Southern Grave

Patients could rarely go home as soon as they were well, particularly in the early years. They had to wait until the conditions were right for planes or ships to get into their district. Sometimes they stayed at the sanatoria, sometimes local accommodation was arranged by the hospital or, as at Caughnawaga and Shubenacadie, by the local Indian agent. Usually, they were sent by air or rail to an intermediate point, such as Churchill or Moose Factory, where they were put up in the military or Indian hospital until further transport was available. Patients returning to the Eastern Arctic might be assembled at Quebec City to await the *C.D. Howe* on its summer run.

Administratively, Health and Welfare was responsible for returning patients to their homes (as it was for bringing them out) and also for their accommodation while awaiting transport home. In the absence of frequent commercial flights, this produced many problems. Different organizations might be involved in flying the patients on the different legs of their journey – private charters, regular commercial flights, RCMP, RCAF, and even the USAF.[1] The charters were far from first class. Medical staff accompanied these flights, and the following is Dr Brian Brett's account of a trip in 1961 when he was in charge of 85 patients going from Mount Hope Airport at Hamilton to Iqaluit.

We chartered a four-engined aircraft and went from Ottawa down to Hamilton to pick them up; and we came back to Ottawa, Robertville, [Kuujjuak], up to the Baffin Island. It was a dreadful trip, just ghastly, for a number of reasons, the first of which was that the person in charge of arranging the flight was overly economic and it was probably the cheapest plane he could get, and it sure looked it. It was in bad shape, and when we stopped at Robertville for oil, for gasoline, they wouldn't give the pilots any because this airline had such a bad name for bad debts. Well, after an awful lot of haggling and my telling the attendants at the pumps that I had 85 sick people, they finally agreed.

Then at one point on the way up the door of the plane opened in mid-air, and I thought this was the most horrendous thing I had ever seen and needed immediate emergency action. I had another doctor and two or three nurses with me, and we somehow got the message across to stay in their seats and buckle up. I went up to the front and told them what had happened and they were pretty nonchalant about the whole thing. And it wasn't the pilot or the co-pilot who came back, it was, I suppose, a cabin-boy. He tried to lasso the door and finally got it, but it wouldn't stay closed and he had to rope it shut. That gives you an idea of the condition of the aircraft. We had one oxygen cylinder, but it was just for one person in case of medical emergency, little thinking we might need it for this!

Anyway, we landed at Iqaluit, and as soon as we got there the police came over and impounded the plane because of the bad debts – a message came from the judge in Yellowknife to impound it. They couldn't have cared less [how we got out again]. We went out by a Nordair DC-3. In those days, I think there were two trips a week up to the north Baffin and we had to wait until the scheduled run got back ... That was a very interesting trip![2]

The patients usually set off on their return trip with some luggage and a label pinned to their parkas, since the transport workers generally knew no Inuktitut and the Inuit knew little or no English or French. The Inuit had virtually no money and no experience or knowledge of the southern transport systems; they were literally in the hands of the transport workers or of the government officer who often accompanied them. Since the two groups also had very different geographical concepts about the land (for instance, the Inuit names for places were not the same as the official names), there were clearly many opportunities for things to go wrong. Sometimes people were dropped off at the wrong place. Often they returned in clothing that was totally inadequate for the conditions of life to which they were returning. In many cases, their families and the local authorities had not been notified of their imminent arrival, and the families might be out on the land in a hunting camp a long way from the settlement.

Clothing was a particular problem. In the late 1940s and through the 1950s, there were many complaints from the settlements and the northern RCMP posts that patients were sent home in clothing suitable only for southern Canada – and certainly not appropriate for former TB patients returning from years in a warm hospital to an igloo in an Arctic winter. For instance, in March 1953 Miss M.E. Hinds, a Northern Affairs teacher at Inukjuak, reported on a man who left

Moose Factory for Akulivik wearing overalls over thick woollen trousers. This clothing was adequate for a journey by plane to Inukjuak, but from there the man had to travel by dog team approximately 300 kilometres to an igloo. Miss Hinds felt that "no patients who live in igloos should be sent back in winter."[3]

In May 1954, after a flight with some Inuit coming in to Winnipeg, G.W. Rowley suggested that Inuit going out to Manitoba should be able to store their northern skin clothing at Churchill Military Hospital, change into southern clothing, and pick up their own clothing on the way back.[4] In January 1955 the RCMP sergeant in charge of the air detachment at Churchill made the same suggestion after flying ten Inuit, including two babies and an 11-year-old girl, from Clearwater Lake Sanatorium, Manitoba, to Churchill, where the temperature was − 32°C. He noted that the women had skirts, women's coats, shoes, and overshoes; and that the men had pants and parkas, and some had overshoes, some boots. Over the week or so that they were quartered in the military hospital while waiting for good weather before flying north to Chesterfield and Baker Lake, six of the group became sick. The sergeant attributed their illness to exposure to the weather. In his report he pointed out the dangers of flying in the North in such clothing because of the risk of exposure in a forced landing, and he demanded that returning Inuit be supplied with adequate native-type clothing and a caribou-hide sleeping bag, at least before flying out of Churchill. He suggested that there be a store of suitable clothing and sleeping bags in Churchill for people awaiting transport farther on.[5]

Evidently, some arrangements about storing clothing at Churchill were made, but slip-ups still occurred. In March 1955 an official in Arctic Division wrote to Major Karpetz at the Churchill Military Hospital about a woman and child who "arrived safely and thrilled with new clothing and toys given her" but who faced a 5-kilometre walk home in a − 36°C temperature without her pants, boots, and parka, and without a hood in which to carry the child, because these had not been sent on with her. The official suggested that the old clothing should be sent back in a box with the patient if necessary.[6]

Eventually, clothing lists for returning patients were circulated to all the sanatoria, instead of leaving the decisions entirely to the uninformed hospital staff. Separate lists were made out for men, women, boys, and girls. They included two sets each of warm and light underwear, trousers, shirts, shoes and/or boots, cardigan, stockings or socks; dresses and tuques or scarves for the women and girls; leather helmets and jeans for the men and boys; and a general issue per person of parka, rubber boots, duffle socks, woollen socks, leather mitts with woollen liners, a sleeping bag, and a kit bag. Babies were to be given a "complete layette" with extra blankets and bunting to protect against the extreme cold. If a patient's northern clothing was still wearable after several years in storage, this was counted against the list and the rest was made up with items made in the hospital by the Inuit women or with donated or store-bought clothes. The hospitals were responsible for providing the clothing, but they billed Northern Administration branch for the cost.

After Walter Rudnicki's Welfare Section was formed in 1956, it kept up the pressure both on its own department for funds and on the INHS to oversee more adequately the provisions made by the hospitals, and the situation gradually improved. (The list circulated in 1957 is given in appendix 4.)[7] Even so, some patients as late as the 1960s arrived home in unsuitable clothes. A patient from Clyde River, who as a teenager was at a southern sanatorium from 1960 to 1963 and returned via a two-week stay in Iqaluit, said she had only a thin coat when she returned. The weather was very cold in Clyde and she had to go by dogsled to her parents' camp out on the land. This lady, who was otherwise very happy about her treatment and was grateful for being cured, told her story through an interpreter:

When she came here they landed on the ice. It was only a small airplane from Iqaluit. Her family wasn't here in camp, they were still out on the land. It seemed like she was – she felt so alone. She didn't know where to go, until a lady from here asked her to come. Then she felt more welcome. They let her borrow a warm coat, warmer, and they took her down to where her parents were. She had to borrow clothes from somebody else because her clothes were too thin. After staying there for four years in the warm weather, when she came here she was very cold.[8]

Besides the clothing allowance, returning TB patients were entitled to a special food ration for six months to a year. This was to enable them to build up their strength during the convalescent period when their physical ability to cope with the demanding Inuit lifestyle and conditions was likely to be marginal. It was in the nature of a medical prescription, similar to post-hospital medicines and vitamin C tablets. But like the clothing, the financing of these rations was the responsibility of Northern Affairs. Health and Welfare was responsible only for the costs of transporting Inuit to and from hospital, for their care, treatment, clothing, and food while in hospital, and for food while awaiting transport to and from hospital. In 1953 the extra rations per person per month were 10 lbs. (4.5 kg) powdered milk, 20 lbs. (9 kg) bannock mix, and 15 lbs. (7 kg) meat or fish.[9]

The families of hunters taken south were also eligible for a standard relief ration, since they were deprived of their food provider.

By 1956, it was realized that the food rations were not sufficiently nutritious, either for the familities or the ex-patients, particularly as items were sometimes substituted at the posts, so a replacement list was issued.[10] The new basic relief ration per person per month consisted of four tins of evaporated milk or ½ lb. (225 g) dried skim or whole milk, nine 28 oz. (800 g) tins of tomatoes or tomato juice (or 1 ascorbic acid tablet a day), 3 lbs. (1.3 kg) lard, 4 lbs. (1.8 kg) fresh or canned meat or fish, 1 lb. (450 g) tea or coffee, 1 lb. (450 g) baking powder, ½ lb. (225 g) salt, and matches and ammunition; and 34 lbs. (15.4 kg) flour plus 4 lbs. (1.8 kg) skim milk powder or 30 lbs. (13.6 kg) oatmeal plus 4 lbs. (1.8 kg) skim milk powder or 35 lbs. (15.9 kg) bannock mix. Those eligible could also have, if requested, 3 lbs. (1.3 kg) of sugar, jam, molasses, syrup, or dried fruit. The new monthly supplementary TB ration was 30–31 multivitamin capsules, 3 lbs. (1.3 kg) rolled dates, 4 lbs. (1.8 kg) skim milk powder, and 3 lbs. (1.3 kg) molasses. As a preventive measure against the spread of TB, families were to be given the additional rations immediately on diagnosis of any member and for six months after the patient's return.

The complicated travel routes not only led to loss of luggage (which was the excuse often given by the medical authorities for a patient's arrival home with inadequate clothing), but they also sometimes led to people being temporarily misplaced. In 1947 the RCMP at Iqaluit complained that returning patients for Kuujjuak, including one Indian, were being delivered via USAF Goose Bay to Iqaluit, where they had to be accommodated at the American base before being sent on to Kuujjuak. In 1953 Coral Harbour reported on some ex-patients from the Camsell hospital and from Winnipeg who were sent to Coral Harbour instead of Igloolik.[11] Such incidents may have been mere inconveniences; some were more serious. One old and confused man from Coppermine was sent by mistake to Aklavik, where he was given refuge in the mission; but not understanding where he was and unable to find his family, he was so unhappy that he committed suicide.[12]

A potentially disastrous return was that of the six-year-old Titus Allooloo, going home from Hamilton to Pond Inlet. He had come out on the *C.D. Howe* in the early 1960s as a suspected TB case, but after spending a few months in the Mountain Sanatorium, he was found to be clear and was fostered out with a local family to await transport home. In December, Allooloo was sent with a group of other patients by bus to Toronto and then by plane to Iqaluit. The

Northern Affairs administrator there assigned him to a family in Apex, the Inuit community just outside Iqaluit proper, but Allooloo did not like the place:

There was quite a bit of drinking going on. I kept running away, running away. Then I was on my own, basically. Every time they found me – the Northern Affairs people – they would drive me back, and I would stay there for a few hours and I would run away ... There were two rehabilitation centres, one for men, one for ladies. That was where I was hanging out, that's where I slept. I was sleeping sometimes under the bed, sometimes on the chairs. That's where I stayed. And the clothing I had was the clothing I had: that was it. I had no change of clothing. Somebody felt sorry for me and gave me a parka. I had a parka then, but I had no luggage, I had nothing else. I don't know what sort of shoes I had, but I had some sort of boots, I think: I can't remember my feet being very cold ... And so I learned how to steal. I was stealing food sometimes, even though there was a place, a cafeteria, where we could go. Sometimes I was stealing money. I wasn't stealing hundreds of dollars, but I was stealing about a dollar, fifty cents, whatever, at that point, to buy candy, and to buy food sometimes.

I was on my own for about six months. I think [the authorities] knew I was not where I was supposed to stay, and that the people there were drinking, that was the reason why I was staying away. And I was supposed to go to school. I attended school sometimes – whenever I could. And once I got to know the city a little bit, the town, I started going to Iqaluit village, which is about three to five miles away from Apex. Hitching a ride and whatever.

Then May that year Indian and Northern Affairs found me and said I'm going home ... There were no scheduled planes at that point, going out of Iqaluit, going up to Pond Inlet. We got into this little single-engine aircraft; there was no room for me to sit, so they put me on top of the luggage. They took off and then there was some problem with the plane so, about an hour out, we turned around and came back to Iqaluit. We slept overnight, then we took off the next day and we travelled all day. I think we landed once, I don't know. We finally landed in Clyde River. Stayed overnight – it was late that day – and then next day we went up to Pond Inlet. My family at that point was not in Pond Inlet. So I stayed in Pond for a little while with the RCMP constable until they came to get me.[13]

Some misplacements may have been due to simple thoughtlessness or callous disregard on the part of the escorts. Rita Burrows, the wife of an Anglican minister in Povungnituk, was at Inukjuak, 240 kilometres to the south, one day in the mid-1960s when she overheard a nurse asking if the baby she was escorting home belonged to anyone at the settlement. Rita Burrows recognized the baby as belonging to a family in Povungnituk and quickly put the nurse to rights. The baby stayed on the plane and eventually reached its mother in Povungnituk.[14]

The Rev. Brian Burrows spent five years in the 1960s as Anglican minister in Povungnituk and was himself treated for TB in the Weston Sanatorium in Toronto in 1965. He considered that the manner in which Inuit returning home were treated reflected the authorities' general lack of respect and responsibility for the people they had ordered to go south for treatment:

They did not think the Eskimo people were worthy of being informed of where they precisely were, and didn't think it important that relatives should be informed, that parents should be told where their children were. There was none of that. The authorities didn't think it important that they should get their names right ... Even when they were written out for them, still they'd get them wrong. Even the Christian names, which they could have got right. And the basic thing behind that, I think, is that they refused to believe that they were people ... I felt that the government should have told them precisely where they were, showed them where it was on a map, and formed some kind of communications.[15]

When a patient died in hospital, Burrows "usually got a call to say, 'Would you tell so-and-so that their baby has died?' or 'their mother has died,' or something like that. Which we did, and prayed with them and helped them in that respect. But there was very little information at all. I'm talking about '62 onward. That was a very, very common thing to happen."[16] Nothing was ever sent directly to the relatives. Instead, messages were relayed through the RCMP, the minister, or some other official. Burrows was firm in his conclusion that the government refused to acknowledge the Inuit as people.

Robert Williamson concurred with Burrows's assessment of the prevailing colonial attitudes and the depersonalizing effect of the powerful whites' disregard for Inuit names and society. Even the channelling of communication through the local whites reinforced a situation in which "the humblest and youngest Hudson's Bay clerk may feel that he has authority over the most dignified and respected old Inuk." Williamson placed the worst examples of bad administration – of the "off-hand, double-standard, rushed way in which the whole medical program was undertaken" – as occurring in the late 1940s and early 1950s. "From the late fifties," he considered, "more and more people were *properly* conveyed, treated and brought home, without getting lost."[17]

Williamson witnessed an incident that typified the situation in the
early years. He was in a hunting camp when a five-year-old boy was
brought home one spring in the early 1950s. Williamson's account of
the boy's return highlights the trauma that must have been experienced by children returning home after years in the South, and by
their parents too. This young boy had been in hospital in Quebec
for several years and had become completely southernized and spoke
only French. When he was fit, he was sent north by stages – in good
southern clothing, and with the best intentions of the hospital staff,
who wanted to get him home in the spring – until he reached a
nursing station not too far from his parents' camp. Here there was a
new nurse, who knew little about the country and had no real
conception of the situation of the boy's family in their hunting camp.
She heard that a mining exploration charter plane was going near
his home and persuaded the party to take the boy along and deliver
him on their way.

The plane duly landed on the frozen lake near the hunting camp.
The prospectors stopped only long enough to put the child out on
the ice far from the shore, and the plane took off, without even
waiting for someone from the camp to come and take the boy or
ensuring that it was the right camp. The family rushed out and picked
up the boy, who was terribly confused and frightened – and cold.
He was wearing a beret, a white shirt with a bow tie, a short-cut
jacket, shorts over lisle stockings, and sandals; and in this outfit he
had been dumped, like so much cargo, on a sheet of ice. As Williamson said,

He was frightened of all these people with their dark brown faces and their
skin clothing, and the smell of the North, you know, of meat and of a different
kind of food. And being nuzzled by these strangers talking loudly, or what
seemed loudly because they were so full of joy, in a totally foreign language,
was not comforting to him. L. picked him up and carried him to the igloo
... and they talked to him about the dogs outside, but he didn't know what
they were saying. And they gave him some morsels of the favourite food
they had, like seal meat, which he ultimately ate and threw up: he ate pilot
biscuits ... By sheer luck, there happened to be staying in that little camp
for a short time a white man with whom he could relate, because he spoke
French, and who could say, "C'est ton papa; c'est ta maman. Tu es à la
maison avec la famille maintenant," and "Be careful of the dogs!" Because
he was a little southern boy in effect, the family were terrified that he would
think the dogs were playthings and they would chew him up.

And that child had a traumatic period of adjustment. He began to sense
quite readily that he was surrounded by love and affection and joy, but it

was a terrible adjustment that he had to go through. I stayed in that camp for some time to help him make the adjustment, interpreting in French and Eskimo for the little boy and for the parents. Well, what would have happened if I hadn't been there? What did happen in many comparable situations where children were brought back north after two or three or four years away, culturally completely southernized, and then dumped unceremoniously, without any preparation either of the child or of the parents, in either hunting camps or ... in shanty towns around the settlements?[18]

Indeed, children presented special problems for the authorities. If they had been in the sanatorium for several years, they often did not want to leave their familiar environment and their friends in order to return to the unknown or barely remembered life up north. The situation of young children sent to Quebec hospitals was particularly awkward. They learned French in the hospital school, lost what Inuit language and skills they had, and then returned to an Inuktitut-speaking family and an English-language school system. They often felt inadequate and were behind their peers in every way, the skills that they had learned down south being very little use to them up north. As one lady from Kuujjuak put it, "I didn't understand Inuktitut any more or English. It's hard trying to talk to your Mom when you don't understand them and they don't know what you're saying. It was hard. You had to find an interpreter to talk to your own family." This patient went out to Roberval when she was "six or seven," stayed there for "two or three years," learned French, and began school. Then she returned home, but she had to go out again. When she came back the second time, she had to begin in kindergarten in the local English school. She recalled, "The other children, five or six years old, were all saying: 'Oh, you're so big and you're so dumb' ... It was hard. I had to work so hard, and used to get so frustrated by it. They picked on me and I had to strike out: 'I'm not dumb!' I spoke French and now I had to learn English all over again. Eventually I skipped grades and caught up with my peers."[19]

Some babies were born in hospital when pregnant women were brought out; a few came with their sick mothers as infants at the breast. The medical staff did not want to expose these babies to infection by keeping them in the sanatoria; but because of the communication and travel problems of the time, the babies could not safely be sent north. In fact, a rule was in force that no infants under six months were to be sent north. Some hospitals, such as the Camsell, set up special nurseries for the infants until they could be sent north to a relative. Perhaps because the IHS had started out as the medical service to the Indians, or because all native peoples were lumped together in the minds of southerners, some doctors used contacts at the Indian Affairs branch to place the children in care on a local Indian reserve. In some cases they may have done so because they lacked help from anyone else and did not know where else to turn. On the reserve, the children were lodgers, sometimes with a family, usually in a ward of an Indian Affairs hospital, where they received only minimal care and little stimulation. Sometimes sympathetic sanatorium staff would unofficially foster a new baby; and there are suggestions that some of these children were subsequently informally adopted, particularly if the mother died in hospital.

In view of the inadequate records in the early days, the difficulties in communication even with the adult patients, the prompt separation of the infant from its unhappy mother, and the death of some of the mothers, there may well have been great difficulty in identifying the families of the infants. It is said that quite a few children were "lost" to the Inuit community this way and remained down south, brought up as part of a southern family.[20] Young children who came out as patients on their own also presented difficulties when they were ready to go home. They, too, were often placed in care on the Indian reserves. One young boy, transferred from Brandon Sanatorium during a flood crisis in 1950, stayed at an Indian residential school for two years until the principal suggested that a more suitable place should be found for him. By then he had lost his language and spoke Cree and English.[21]

In 1956 the Northern Administration and Lands branch, as part of its normal Inuit administration, began to organize foster-home placement for Inuit children who were orphans or were disabled and required special care which their families could not provide.[22] As Rudnicki's fledgling Welfare Section gathered more staff and information about the Inuit patients scattered across the country, they began to intervene with the medical authorities to introduce formal foster-home care for the hospital babies. In March 1958, Betty Marwood met with the Children's Aid Society (CAS) of Hamilton, with Dr Hayward (the medical superintendent of the Lady Willingdon Indian Hospital at Oshweken on the Brantford reserve, which had been caring for the well babies from the Mountain Sanatorium), and with Dr Ewart, the medical superintendent of the sanatorium.[23] By June, the CAS had agreed to take responsibility for placing the children in temporary foster homes. Dr Ewart's subsequent circular to his staff set out the conditions for foster home placement for the Inuit babies:

- Only healthy babies would be placed and then only if they would be remaining in a home for a reasonable length of time.
- The foster parents would be advised by the CAS that there was no prospect of adoption.
- Newborns would remain at the sanatorium for a minimum of 14 days.
- The Welfare Section would be advised of all placements, which would be arranged by the Social Service Department of the hospital and the CAS.[24]

By July, the last two Inuit children from the Oshweken hospital had been placed in foster homes in Hamilton to await their mothers' repatriation home.[25] Thereafter, there was a steady trickle of letters from the CAS to Rudnicki recording the fostering-out of new babies.

Similar arrangements were made with the CAS of western Manitoba to care for children from the Brandon Sanatorium, and with the INHS in The Pas for children from Clearwater Lake. In Montreal, Inuit children had been lodged at the Indian hospital on the Caughnawaga reserve, and Marwood persuaded the Protestant Children's Homes in Montreal to arrange foster care for these children. This brought much relief to the lone and overworked Indian Affairs doctor at Caughnawaga, who was responsible for all the Indians and Inuit coming into and leaving Montreal, as well as those on the reserve.[26]

The Travellers' Aid Society, alerted to the difficulties of Inuit passing through Montreal, set up a service to meet their trains or planes and to help them make their connections. Through a member of this organization, a series of transit foster homes was set up in Huntingdon, a small town near Montreal, for adults waiting to go home. Here they could live in homes instead of an institution and walk about the village more safely and easily than in Montreal. The townsfolk became very protective of the patients and interested in helping them. When one Inuk died before he could return home, the village gave him a magnificent funeral. Photographs of the funeral were carried up north by the nurse on the Eastern Arctic Patrol, where they were passed on to Betty Marwood to give to the man's widow. Before handing over the photos, Marwood and her interpreter consulted the widow's mother about the situation. The mother was very pleased that her daughter would receive the photos because, although she had been told that her husband was dead, she did not believe it. Many people had gone out to hospital and the families never knew what had happened; then several years later they came back. So her daughter could not get on with her life, she could not let her husband go, because she thought he was coming back. The pictures would prove to her that he had actually died, and she would be able to let him go.[27]

Many patients died in the sanatoria, particularly during the early years of the program. At that time, the disease was often far advanced when the cases were found, the effective drug treatments were not yet available, and the psycho-social support services were not in place to help the patients fight their illness. Theoretically, when a patient died, the hospital notified the IHS, and the IHS notified Northern Affairs, which in turn notified its contact in the patient's community (usually, the local RCMP or missionary), who told the relatives. But many messages never got through. The patient never returned, and the families were simply left wondering what had happened.[28] As Brian Burrows said, even when the news did arrive, it was only a bald statement that so-and-so had died. There were no details about the cause of death, no information about the burial, no letter of explanation or condolence – just a radio call or cable or, later, a telephone call through an official.[29]

The patients were buried at Northern Affairs' expense in paupers' graves in a local cemetery. Often they were buried on Indian reserves, as at Caughnawaga or Stony Plain; often in municipal cemeteries by regular funeral homes.[30] But the relatives were not told where and the graves were not marked, though most cemetery authorities have records of the location of each body. Burrows is now a minister in Hamilton and has several times been asked by Inuit searching for the graves of their relatives to say prayers in Inuktitut at the Inuit graves in the Hamilton municipal cemetery. "Because," as he said, "in their mind they didn't know where they were. So they were still, as it were, unburied even though a service had been taken. But, of course, it would be in English and they weren't present." He thinks that the bodies should have been sent back up north, as they are now, despite the expense. Otherwise "somebody goes and disappears and never comes back, and you have no sort of tangible proof that your loved one died."[31]

To the Inuit, it was often as though a child had been kidnapped and lost for ever. And their inability to do anything about it except ask the "kidnappers" for news (which, if it came at all, came slowly, rarely, and sparsely) must have made the anguish even worse. But the Inuit did not give up seeking news of their lost relatives, and the Welfare Section received many letters asking about them. Many patients in hospital also wrote to the section, worried about their families and begging to go home. Some of these letters expressed appreciation of news given by a welfare official or of help given by the medical staff; others were from people asking to be sent – or not sent – to another hospital. In the period 1956–63, at least 20 per cent of the adult population of the Eastern Arctic wrote to the Welfare Service specifically in connection with the TB hospitalization program.[32]

As the section grew and became a division, more translators were hired and syllabic typewriters acquired, and the welfare workers spent many hours answering queries, explaining why it was necessary for someone to go out to hospital, and passing on reports and news. The following letter was written by Robert Williamson in February 1959. The names have been changed to protect the family's privacy.

Dear Joe,

Mr Lee asked me to write to you because of your fear about your son going out to hospital. I am sorry that you were away when the "C.D. Howe" was in [your settlement], because then you could have talked to the social worker who would have explained why the doctor wanted your son to go to hospital. Your son's TB is not bad, but it is such that if it is not treated it will get worse. In 1957, when the doctor saw Don, he had a slight shadow on his lung. The doctor hoped this would get better by itself so he did not advise that your son go out to hospital. Last summer when the doctor saw that this was getting worse and not better as he had hoped he advised that your son go to hospital for treatment.

We know that it takes a long time for people to recover from TB, but this is something that cannot be helped. We also know that if people are not getting better and wait too long to get treatment then they will die. Sometimes people think they are being kept in hospital longer than necessary, but this is not so. The doctors do not want people to stay in hospital too long. It is only that sometimes people may appear well to others who are not doctors, but the doctors know that they are not completely better, they only appear so. The doctor wants to be sure that they are completely better before letting them go home.

It is a long way from [your settlement] to Mountain San. and many people do not realize that there are times when it is difficult to arrange for transportation for people to return to their homes. For example, as you know the "C.D. Howe" only goes up north once a year. It leaves the south early in the summer and has many places to stop before it gets to [your settlement] ... If a person is ready to leave the hospital in the spring returning on the ship might be the easiest way for him to go home. If it is possible the people are always sent by plane, but if not they have to wait for the ship.

It is also true that some people in the old days got better without the doctor's help, but many people died whom a doctor could have saved. It is also true that some people did die after operations even though the doctor does his best to prevent this, but these are only the people who are very sick before the doctor operates, and many more people get better after operations than die.

I am very sorry that Joy has been worrying about Ann so much that she is losing weight. Had you only known you could have asked Mr Lee to find out how Ann was. When Mr Lee told us about Joy worrying we wrote to the doctor. He says that Ann is getting along very well in hospital and even though she would rather be home she is not unhappy there. She is getting better and if she continues to do as well as she has in the last few months she will be ready to go home in the spring. Please try not to worry about your daughter and trust us to return her to you as soon as she is cured of her TB. This we will also do with Don. Ann is going to school while in hospital, and you can be proud as to how well she is doing.

Because we know that you and other Eskimos are worried about relatives in hospital, we are sending reports home as often as we can. We will ask Mr Lee to let you know from time to time how Don is getting along. If you wish to write to me my address is ...[33]

As facilities, cash flow, and travel improved in the North, and as more Inuit became accustomed to southern ways and were able to travel south on their own account, some began to search for the graves of their relatives or to approach their local MLA for help in getting information about them. Eventually, in January 1989, a program was set up by the Government of the Northwest Territories to help search for the missing relatives. Called the Medical Patient Search Project, it covered Inuit, Dene, and other northern native people.[34] The project staff contacted the provincial offices of vital statistics and the cemetery and hospital authorities in towns to which northern native patients had been sent. Searches were also made of church and cemetery records, death certificates, and, where possible, hospital records. The searches were difficult even for accredited government officials. Many of the sanatoria are now closed or converted to other uses, and the patients' records have been transferred or destroyed. Moreover, provincial offices of vital statistics require specific identifying information, the records of which are sometimes inaccurate or lost.

In December 1989 the project officer, Jo MacQuarrie, helped Charlie Crow, the MLA for Sanikiluaq, in his search for 18 missing people about whom he had been asked by members of his community. Together they went to Moosonee, Montreal, and Hamilton, searching hospital, Anglican church, and cemetery records, and located 12 of the missing people, including four of Crow's own relatives. By May

1990, the project staff had received requests for help from 63 families and had completed 45 searches, reuniting one man with his family in the Eastern Arctic and providing information on the deaths of 44. In the summer and fall of 1990 a media campaign of the northern communities gave families a final opportunity to request searches before the project closed down the following spring. This resulted in a further 17 requests. In all, by April 1991, 80 requests had been received (regarding 64 Inuit patients, 15 Dene, and one other) and information and records had been found and forwarded to the families of 71 of the lost patients. Although the project closed down in April 1991, the same search mechanism and communication channels are being used by the NWT Department of Health to investigate the cases remaining on the books and any other requests for information that may be made.

Meanwhile, a movement has been growing to erect memorials in the various burial places to patients whose bodies lie in the unmarked graves.[35] In Alberta, a cairn was erected in 1990 at St Albert's Aboriginal Cemetery, on the outskirts of St Albert, to commemorate the Indian and Inuit patients who died at the Charles Camsell Hospital between 1946 and 1966 and were buried in this cemetery. The cemetery was originally associated with an adjoining United Church Indian residential school, and DIAND had employed students from the school to dig the graves. The school closed in the early 1970s, and in 1979 the abandoned and neglected cemetery was turned over to the city of St Albert by the federal government. The city officials wanted to build a memorial to those buried there, but could find no grave plan or records at either DIAND or the provincial government, so the site was tidied up, the grave mounds levelled, and the few remaining nameless markers removed.

Then a group of former staff from the Charles Camsell Hospital became involved: the matron, Elva Taylor; Dr Otto Schaefer; a nurse, Maxine LeClair, who remembered accompanying patients to the cemetery for the funerals of their friends; and Don McBride, a teacher at the Camsell hospital, 1957–62, who went on to be administrator of the Indian residential school, 1962–68. McBride and his staff at the school had in fact kept a record of the burials and had passed them to the Anglican chaplain. Now the records were combined with diagrams from the city landscape planner, John Beedle, who had levelled the site, and McBride recreated the plot plan to show the locations of individual graves. The group succeeded in getting funds from the Alberta and Northwest Territories governments to raise the cairn, which lists the names, places of birth, and dates of death of 98 Indian, Métis, and Inuit patients. Roman Catholic patients from the Camsell were buried in the Stony Plain Indian Reserve Cemetery west of Edmonton, served by Our Lady of Mercy Mission, where records are sketchy and graves still unmarked.

In Hamilton a similar movement is under way to put up a granite monument in the city's Woodland Cemetery, where most of those who died in the Mountain Sanatorium are buried. This project was started in 1989 by the city's director of cemeteries, Chester Orzel, who examined the cemetery records of the 1950s and 1960s and drew up a list of 33 Inuit patients who were buried there between 1952 and 1963.[36] He also has a grave plan, showing where each person is buried, though the graves themselves have only wooden markers. Two – in one case, three – bodies lie one above the other in one grave, though in separate caskets and separated with earth. This is a common practice in city cemeteries, whether in purchased family plots or paupers' graves. Although Orzel is now retired, he has continued to work on this project and has designed a granite memorial based on carvings which were made by the patients while in the sanatorium and which are now in the lobby of the Chedoke Hospital (as the old Mountain Sanatorium is now called). Orzel has tried to get funds for the memorial from the city of Hamilton and the NWT government; and the city, in its turn, has applied to DIAND, which is "very sympathetic" to the project.[37]

Clearwater Lake, The Pas, was the third centre designated by Dr Moore in 1955 for Inuit TB patients. There, an RCMP officer, Corporal Mel Hollett, has worked to identify the gravesites of patients who died while in the sanatorium or at St Anthony's. Hollett was inspired by an Inuk special constable in Iqaluit with whom he had worked, the brother of one of the missing patients. By searching the records of the town office and the church registries, he has put together a list of patients, with their ages and dates of birth and burial. Anglicans were generally buried in the Lakeside Cemetery, and Roman Catholics in the Riverside Cemetery, but some patients were buried in the Mile Six Cemetery on the Métis Indian Reserve nearby. Hollett's efforts to get individual stones to mark the graves has been taken on by a group of citizens of The Pas, who are seeking funding from the NWT Department of Health to complete the project.[38]

Perhaps eventually the graves of all the Inuit who died and were buried so far away from their homes and families will be identified by more personal and respectful markers than the wooden stakes with grave plot numbers that, even in the best-kept cemeteries, are all that mark them now.

CHAPTER TEN

The 1960s:

New Measures in the Northwest Territories

In 1961 the Indian and Northern Health Service was renamed Medical Services branch, but its Arctic component continued to be known as the Northern Health Service (NHS), and through the 1960s the program of surveys, immunization, and evacuation to southern hospitals continued to be the mainstay of its fight against TB. More nursing stations and health centres were opened, and links were developed between the small northern hospitals and the medical schools in the South which supplied visiting specialists.

The Department of National Health and Welfare was legally responsible for health services to the Inuit in the Northwest Territories and northern Quebec, and since Newfoundland's entry into Confederation in 1949, it had tacitly accepted responsibility for those in Labrador by helping to fund their hospitalization. But the exact arrangements between the federal government and the three lower levels of government varied somewhat. About two-thirds of the Inuit live in the Northwest Territories. In the 1960s they made up over one-third of the population of the territory. Here, the Medical Services branch continued to supply medical services to the whole of the population, receiving funding from the NWT government for those given to non-natives. The five-year plan it developed in 1961 set out three levels of service, depending on the size and accessibility of the communities.[1]

The first level of service was for tiny communities of a few people, where rudimentary health training and a small salary would be given to one resident health-care worker and the community would be "visited but rarely by a physician or nurse." The second level was for larger settlements located on established communication lines; it consisted of a nursing station of the type already in operation in a number of settlements, from which nurses could visit outlying families and be in radio contact with a physician. The third level applied to the largest settlements, towns, or regional centres, which were served by resident physicians and dentists and had one or more hospitals.

The existing facilities in Inuit country in 1961 were listed as:

- five hospitals, at Inuvik, Iqaluit, Chesterfield Inlet, Rankin Inlet, and Pangnirtung;
- eight nursing stations, at Aklavik, Cambridge Bay, Coppermine, Spence Bay, Tuktoyaktuk, Baker Lake, Arviat, and Cape Dorset;
- four clinics (which provided out-patient treatment, a public-health unit, and a physician), at Inuvik, Rankin Inlet, Iqaluit, and Pangnirtung; and
- seven health stations (an accommodation hut for visiting medical staff), at Bathurst Inlet, Gjoa Haven, Perry River, Sachs Harbour, Arctic Bay, Padloping, and Pond Inlet.

These facilities were all operated by the NHS, except for the mission hospitals at Chesterfield Inlet and Pangnirtung and the nickel mine hospital and clinic at Rankin Inlet.

The 1961 plan called for 14 new facilities and 73 new staff (including 32 native health workers) to be in place throughout the Northwest Territories by 1966. In Inuit country, the planned facilities were a larger hospital at Iqaluit, four nursing stations (at Coral Harbour, Padloping, Arctic Bay, and Pond Inlet), and six health stations or MO's residences (at Pelly Bay, Cambridge Bay, Read Island, Repulse Bay, Igloolik, and Port Burwell). By 1969, these plans were reported to have been "quite satisfactorily implemented."[2]

People suffering from cancer, tuberculosis, or severe mental illness, and those without money were entitled to free investigation and treatment, and transportation to the nearest adequate medical facility. In 1961, J. Waldo Monteith, the minister of health and welfare, estimated the average cost of treatment of a person with TB to be $3,500 to $5,000 a year, or $3,500 to $15,000 a case, excluding transportation expenses, which could run as high as $2,000.[3] Thus, the programs were far from cheap. As might be expected, the overall cost of medical care for the Inuit had also risen from the measly sum of $6.46 per person in 1944–45. In 1961–62 the annual cost was $291 per person.[4]

Persuading physicians, particularly specialists, to work in the professional isolation of the Far North was always difficult, and vacancies often remained unfilled for many months.[5] To help interest young doctors in service in the North, and to expand their professional knowledge, the Canadian Association of Medical Students and

Table 13
Yield of Case-Finding Activities among Inuit, 1974–75

	No. of examinations	No. of active cases found	No. of examinations per case
X-ray surveys	10,247	2	5,123
Referred films	14,309	44	325
Sputum surveys	11,339	19	597

Source: S. Grzybowski, K. Styblo, and E. Dorken, "Tuberculosis in Eskimos," *Tubercle* 57, no. 4, supp. (1976): s9, s39.

Interns, in collaboration with the NHS and the universities, arranged a summer program for 70 senior medical students in 1967.[6] The students came from every Canadian medical school, and together with 20 experienced faculty members, they spent three weeks in the Far North: ten days in Inuvik for lectures, films, discussions and ward-rounds; seven days of small-group fieldwork in 12 Indian or Inuit settlements (including Aklavik, Coppermine, Cambridge Bay, Tuktoyaktuk, and Spence Bay); and three days at Edmonton for summation and evaluation. It later became the practice for some medical schools to send their senior students north to work with the NHS for a period.

Through the 1960s, large-scale TB diagnostic techniques moved from a reliance on x-ray surveys to include more Mantoux tests and, from 1967 on, mass sputum surveys.[7] This resulted in more accurate case-finding and a (temporary) apparent increase in incidence. BCG vaccination, which had been carried out sporadically since the late 1940s, was introduced on a large scale in 1965, when it was routinely given to all newborns and to people who had a negative Mantoux reaction even if they had previously been vaccinated. Active case-finding in the Keewatin had lagged behind that in the Baffin and Western Arctic, but after an outbreak of TB in Arviat in 1963 (when 82 new cases were found in six months in a community of only 329 people)[8] more attention was paid to this area. In 1967, for instance, 4,000 chest x-rays, 1,605 Mantoux tests, and 478 BCG vaccinations were carried out in the Keewatin.[9]

Besides the mass x-ray and sputum surveys that were carried out annually – or, in some settlements, twice a year – the local nursing stations x-rayed patients seeking medical advice for symptoms or people referred by the NHS centre in Edmonton because of inactive TB, close contact with patients, et cetera. This proved to be the most efficient method for discovering active cases of tuberculosis. The 1974–75 figures show the relative efficiency (see table 13).

Table 14
Inuit Patients Receiving Treatment for Tuberculosis, 1966–74[1]

	1966–68	1969–71	1972–74
Average number of patients in treatment	259	323	164
% treated as out-patients	54%	82%	86%
Average number on preventive drugs	52	539	931

Source: Statistics Canada, tuberculosis statistics, morbidity and mortality, 1966–74, cats. 83–206 and 82–212.

[1] Three-year averages and percentages calculated by author.

Home chemotherapy and chemoprophylaxis also became more widely used. Chemotherapy was continued for a time at home for patients discharged from sanatoria, and from the late 1960s on, it was used for an increasing proportion of newly diagnosed patients. Chemoprophylaxis, or a preventive course of drugs, was given to close contacts considered to be poor risks, to people having a positive reaction on a tuberculin test, to people with inactive tuberculosis, and to patients who had regained a normal sputum analysis following a course of chemotherapy. In 1966, the first year these statistics were recorded by Statistics Canada, only 20 per cent of the patients under treatment were out-patients and a further eight people were receiving preventive treatment. In 1974, 90 per cent of the patients were being treated as out-patients and a further 760 people were receiving preventive treatment. The three-year averages for the relevant years are shown in table 14. The medications were given directly to the patients by the nurse or community health worker; or, in the case of children, by a teacher at their school. When introduced carefully into a community, with good explanations, the medications were well accepted and proved very effective in helping to prevent further outbreaks such as the one at Arviat.[10]

The drop in the number of patients also made it easier for the NHS to cut down on the number of hospitals to which Inuit were sent. In the early 1960s the NHS stopped sending patients to the Mountain Sanatorium in Hamilton (which had previously been the most frequented sanatorium for Inuit from the Eastern Arctic) and gathered all the TB patients in southern Ontario at the Weston Sanatorium in Toronto. In 1968 the NHS reported that all its TB patients, both Indian and Inuit, were in ten hospitals: the Charles Camsell; the Alberta Sanatorium; the Alberta Hospital, Edmonton; Faraud Hospital, Rae; Inuvik General Hospital; Ninette Sanatorium; Weston Sanatorium; Moose Factory Indian Hospital; St Luke's, Pangnirtung; and the D.A. Stewart Centre, Winnipeg.[11]

Table 15
Inuit Tuberculosis Morbidity, 1961–65 (Rates per 100,000 Population)

| | Hospital admissions | | | | | Patients in treatment | |
| | First admission (incidence) | | | Total | | In hospital | % of TB patient population |
Year	Number	Rate[1]	Readmissions	Number	Rate[1]		
1961	182	1,538	81	263	2,222	248	4
1962	177	1,496	67	244	2,062	255	5
1963	231	1,952	112	343	2,898	299	7
1964	92	777	53	145	1,225	209	5
1965	106	896	53	159	1,343	170	5

Sources: Statistics Canada, tuberculosis statistics, morbidity and mortality, cat. 83–206.
[1] Rates calculated by author.

As the permanent land-based medical services increased, the dependence on the annual *C.D. Howe* patrol decreased, and in 1969 the medical patrol was discontinued. Air survey teams, using DC-3 aircraft on skis in the spring and Twin Otter float-planes in the fall, supplemented the permanent land-based staff. As well, some regular commercial flights were by then available, making medical evacuations easier.[12]

During the 1960s and 1970s, the medical programs began to bear real fruit in statistical terms. The numbers in the sanatoria and the death rate began to decline markedly. The incidence, after remaining (in real terms) around 1 per cent of the population, had dropped dramatically by the mid-1970s; and the average length of time in hospital fell to 18.3 months by the early 1960s and to 2.9 months by the early 1970s.[13] Morbidity and mortality statistics from 1961 on are given in tables 15 to 18. Figure 1 shows the decline in morbidity from 1960 to 1982. Statistics Canada mortality data are based on death certificates. They cannot be relied on after 1973, when the provinces dropped ethnic origin from the requirements on death certificates. Although ethnic origin continued to be reported by the Northwest Territories, the completeness of the information (shown by the "% total origin not stated" column in table 17) varied from year to year. Medical Services branch, however, continued to record statistics on its patients by ethnic origin and in 1968 computerized its TB case records. This resulted, it was said, in more accurate statistical data.[14]

This measure also led to a more efficient follow-up of patients and to the discovery that 20 per cent of the population had old inactive TB and, indeed, needed to be followed up regularly in case of

Table 16
Inuit Tuberculosis Morbidity, 1966–90 (Rates per 100,000 Population)

	Reported cases					Patients in treatment		
	New active (incidence)			Total		In hospital	Out-patient	% of TB patient population
Year	Number	Rate[1]	Reactivated	Number	Rate[1]			
1966	119	1,005	23	142	1,200	180	46	2
1967	136	1,149	30	166	1,403	76	126	2
1968	121	1,022	32	153	1,293	103	247	3
1969	161	1,360	32	193	1,631	97	277	3
1970	105	887	25	130	1,098	36	281	3
1971	87	496	20	107	610	42	236	3
1972	50	285	20	70	399	25	164	2
1973	49	279	14	63	359	32	138	2
1974	39	222	13	52	296	13	120	2
1975	41	234	10	51	291	Total =	142[2]	2
1976	27	154	3	30	171	Total =	119[2]	2
1977	20	114	12	32	182	–	–	–
1978	23	131	8	31	177	–	–	–
1979	12	68	7	19	108	–	–	–
1980	17	97	2	19(20)[3]	108	–	–	–
1981	19	82	5	24(22)[3]	108	–	–	–
1982	28	121	10	38	164	–	–	–
1983	39	168	9	48	207	–	–	–
1984	7	30	6	13	56	–	–	–
1985	18	78	4	22	95	–	–	–
1986	17	73	6	23	99	–	–	–
1987	6	26	1	7(12)[3]	30	–	–	–
1988	24	103	2	26(21)[3]	112	–	–	–
1989	25	108	9	34	147	–	–	–
1990	5	22	3	8	34	–	–	–

Sources: Statistics Canada, tuberculosis statistics, morbidity and mortality, cats. 83–206 and 82–212, and health reports, cat. 82–003s10.
[1] Rates calculated by author.
[2] Patients under treatment were not reported after 1976.
[3] Figures in parentheses are the revised figures given in Health Reports 4, no. 2, 1992.

breakdown. The reactivation of old inactive tuberculosis seems to be a greater problem among the Inuit than in the white population. It certainly was in the 1960s and 1970s. In contrast to the usual pattern among whites, among Inuit the risk of reactivation was fairly small during the first few years after treatment, but it increased steadily as time went on, reaching a peak after ten years. Fortunately, in about 80 per cent of the reactivated cases, the bacilli were fully susceptible to all three standard drugs. The average annual risk of reactivation

Table 17
Inuit Tuberculosis Mortality by Certified Number of Deaths, 1961–89

Year	Canada					Northwest Territories	
		Origin not stated					% total
	Total	No.	% total[1]	All others	Known Inuit	Known Inuit	origin not stated[1]
1961	780	189	24	585	6	5	10
1962	798	239	30	548	11	9	7
1963	760	221	29	531	8	5	11
1964	675	213	32	458	4	3	0
1965	695	209	30	479	7	7	0
1966	675	212	31	460	3	3	0
1967	658	194	29	460	4	4	0
1968	640	203	32	435	2	2	0
1969	560	190	34	366	4	4	0
1970	586	241	41	343	2	2	33
1971	511	248	49	260	3	2	50
1972	468	179	38	283	6	3	17
1973	442	208	47	231	3	2	0
1974	337	302	90	31	4	4	17
1975	278	264	95	14	0	0	100
1976	264	255	97	7	2	2	0
1977	260	253	97	5	2	2	0
1978	220	211	96	8	1	1	25
1979	202	196	97	6	0	0	0
1980	188	181	96	7	0	0	25
1981	205	203	99	1	1	1	0
1982	197	194	98	3	0	0	50
1983	202	198	98	3	1	1	67
1984	182	174	96	4	4	4	20
1985	206	206	100	0	0	0	100
1986	182	181	99	0	1	1	67
1987	155	155	100	0	0	0	0
1988	160	160	100	0	0	0	0
1989	188	186	99	1	1	1	33

Source: Statistics Canada, Canadian Centre for Health Information, *Mortality Deaths (Tuberculosis) by Ethnic Origin*, custom tabulation, 1992.
[1] Percentages calculated by author.

in the late 1960s was 1.3 per cent. It dropped to 0.75 per cent by 1974, but this was still considerably higher than in the white population, where the risk was around 0.2 per cent.[15]

As the numbers of new active cases declined, the proportion of reactivated cases (which stemmed, of course, from the active cases of up to a decade or so earlier) among the patient population

Table 18
Inuit Tuberculosis Mortality Rates, 1961–72 (Rates per 100,000 Population)

Year	According to Statistics Canada		According to Medical Services Branch	
	Annual	Average[1]	Annual	Average[1]
1961	51		70	
1962	93		82	
1963	68		51	
1964	34	62	35	60
1965	59		60	
1966	25		0	
1967	34		10	
1968	17	34	3	18
1969	34		3	
1970	17		3	
1971	17		0	
1972	34	26	3	2

Sources: Statistics Canada, Canadian Centre for Health Information, *Mortality Deaths (Tuberculosis) by Ethnic Origin*, custom tabulation, 1992; and S. Grzybowski, K. Styblo, and E. Dorken, "Tuberculosis in Eskimos," *Tubercle* 57, no. 4, supp. (1976), from Medical Services Branch's data on Northwest Territories.
[1] Averages calculated by author.

increased, levelling off at around one-third of all cases. The proportion of reactivated cases for 1960–83 was as follows:

1960–62	11.2%
1963–65	10.1%
1966–68	14.6%
1969–71	24.0%
1972–74	30.3%
1975–77	18.5%
1978–80	31.0%
1981–83	37.5%[16]

Although these figures relate only to Inuit in the Northwest Territories, they show how important it is for former TB patients to have medical check-ups even ten or fifteen years after a "cure."

Despite the different pattern of reactivations in Inuit and white patients, there seem to be no real clinical or radiological differences in the disease between the two groups.[17] In the 1970s the proportion of far-advanced disease in Inuit patients, which had been very high

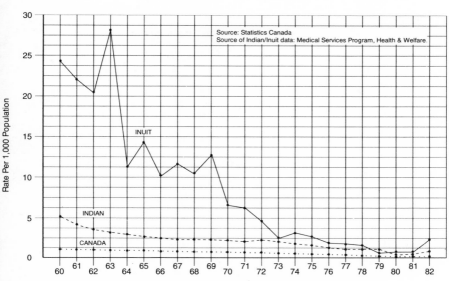

Figure 1   Tuberculosis Rates, 1960–82 (New and Reactivated Cases)

in the 1950s, declined to well below that for the Canadian population as a whole (4 per cent compared with 20 per cent), while the proportion of minimal disease found increased accordingly (61 per cent compared with 35 per cent). This probably reflects the results of the intensive case-finding program among the Inuit and Indians, which is absent in the rest of the population. The average age of the patients also gradually increased. In the early 1960s, 44 per cent of Inuit TB patients in hospital were 14 years of age or younger. In the late 1960s this group made up only 24 per cent of the patients under treatment (including out-patients), and by the 1970s it was only 12 per cent (see table 19).

While the NHS concentrated on the physical aspects of disease in the North, the Welfare Section at Northern Affairs continued to try to pick up the pieces. In 1956 Rudnicki put forward an ambitious five-year plan for the development of welfare services in the North-west Territories and northern Quebec. This involved:

- the gradual decentralization of administration to three regional centres at Fort Smith, Churchill, and Iqaluit;
- the phased-in application of services to all residents of the area;
- the development of rehabilitation centres at Aklavik, Churchill, and Iqaluit;
- the development of subsidiary units at 10 other settlements in the territories, seven of them in the Arctic;

Table 19
Percentage Distribution of Inuit Tuberculosis Patients by Age Group, 1961–76

| Age group | % of hospital patient population 1961–65 (pop. 1180)[1] | % of patients receiving treatment (in hospital or as out-patients)[1] | |
		1966–71, omitting 1968[2] (pop. 1397)	1972–76 (pop. 753)
0–4	18	9	2
5–14	24	15	10
15–24	17	22	17
25–34	15	19	19
35–44	12	13	22
45–54	8	10	13
55–64	5	7	9
65–74	2	3	5
75+	1	1	2

Source: Statistics Canada, tuberculosis statistics, morbidity and mortality, cats. 83–206 and 82–212.
[1] Percentages calculated by author. Numbers may not add up because of rounding.
[2] Statistics Canada figures for 1968 were based on out-patients only.

- additional funding for such items as transit centres, foster and boarding home care, northern allowances, clothing and sleeping bags, food, travel for Inuit, sanitary supplies, resettlement, and a children's receiving home;
- an increase in staff from 10 in the fiscal year 1956–57 to 59 in 1961–62; and
- an increase in budget from $357,210 in 1956–57 to $868,940 in 1961–62.[18]

The Welfare Section increased in size and in 1959 became a division under the Northern Administration branch (NAB), which replaced the Northern Administration and Lands branch that year. Nonetheless, Rudnicki had considerable difficulty in achieving his aims. He had the impression that his planning was considered subversive and that he himself was viewed as an activist, going beyond his mandate.[19] There never seemed to be money available from Treasury Board at the same time for both the capital expenditure needed for the new buildings and equipment and for the staff needed to run the facilities, and he was driven to devise creative solutions to the problems he and his workers saw. For instance, in the absence of any surety of adequate transit facilities for patients on the way home from hospital – or, when they arrived there, of housing in which they could make a reasonable adjustment to the severe northern environment – Rudnicki purchased $60,000 of eiderdown sleeping bags to be issued to patients returning north. He thought this was regarded as remarkable licence, but as he said, it "was just a sort of low-income housing program. They provided a very effective support ... reduced the relapse rate."[20]

By January 1962, although Rudnicki still had neither the staff nor the degree of decentralization originally planned, some progress had been made.[21] Rehabilitation centres were in operation at Inuvik and Iqaluit, and children's receiving homes at Churchill, Iqaluit, Baker Lake, and Fort Smith; homes for the aged were operating in Chesterfield and Aklavik;[22] transit centres for people coming from or going to hospital were operating at Aklavik, Inuvik, Cambridge Bay, Kuujjuak, Iqaluit, and Churchill; 137 prefabricated houses had been built for indigent and medically disabled families, mainly in the Arctic District; an Inuktitut language magazine was being published, and translation services were provided for most Inuit in hospital; the family allowances store-credit system had been replaced with payment by cheque as in the rest of the country; and new policies and procedures regarding relief and child welfare had been worked out. The plans for 1962 centred on increasing the effectiveness of the existing programs and developing ways to involve local communities in as many aspects of the work as possible so that they could play a more direct and vital role in the administration of their own affairs.

The NAB programs, like the medical programs, were, of course, initiated in Ottawa by southern civil servants with virtually no direct input from the Inuit. But the work of the Welfare Division naturally involved a lot of contact with individuals from the Inuit community, and consequently the staff were perhaps more sensitive to the feelings and aspirations of the people than were the medical staff, most of whom had a much more technical and intermittent relationship with them and met them almost exclusively in the authoritarian-dependent context of the doctor-patient situation.

One of the programs that NAB brought to fruition was the setting-up of the rehabilitation centres, which were mainly to help TB patients who were no longer strong enough to follow their arduous traditional way of life. Typically, the subject was under discussion for years before anything concrete emerged. As early as 1951, the NA&L branch's files are full of memos, reports of interdepartmental meetings, and suggestions and countersuggestions about the various needs of convalescent Inuit TB patients and others who required residential support and perhaps vocational training but not medical treatment.[23] It seems to have been clearly recognized that there was a need for supportive programs both for patients while in hospital and for convalescents. But sorting through the multiplicity of jurisdictions, financial responsibilities, and divergent views on what would be best for the Inuit and, possibly, the hidden agenda of the various groups involved, made progress in practical terms rather slow.

Both the Roman Catholic and the Anglican missions had set up small units or industrial homes alongside their Arctic hospitals, mainly for the care of the local old or infirm. But they were loth to expand these facilities, having suffered financial losses with them as a result of the government's miserly annual rate of $200 per person.[24] NANR officials were full of pious words but were still apparently in their lethargic prewar mode. The doctors were adamant that some place must be found to accommodate patients who no longer needed hospital care but were considered to be unfit to return immediately to the rigours of the North. There was even a suggestion that an Inuit colony should be set up near some large southern town where the convalescents could receive suitable job training and learn to adjust to the southern way of life.[25]

In March 1953, in the face of opposition both from missionaries and from Northern Affairs, Dr Moore pushed through a plan to set up an Inuit convalescent centre for male patients from the Camsell hospital at Driftpile, Alberta, on an experimental basis, and two patients were duly sent there.[26] One was a paraplegic, the other nearly blind, and no training staff were available for them at the centre, which was a primarily Indian community. Both men were very unhappy at Driftpile, threatening to "walk out" and asking to go home to Coppermine. By June it was clear even to Dr Moore that this was not a suitable arrangement, and he asked Northern Affairs if the men could be transferred to the rehabilitation centre proposed for Aklavik. The Aklavik centre, however, was not scheduled to open until 1954 (and, in fact, was never built), so arrangements were made with the Department of Veterans Affairs to take the patients at the Rideau Health and Occupational Centre in Ottawa. Judging from the correspondence, this also seems to have been in the nature of an experiment, paid for by Northern Affairs at a daily rate of $7.50, plus a $7.00-a-month comforts allowance.[27]

After some delay, the two men were duly flown to Ottawa, but the families were not informed. In November 1953 the Rev. Sperry wrote to the Charles Camsell Hospital inquiring about the whereabouts of one of the patients on behalf of his family, who wanted him home. The family had received a letter from him saying how homesick and unhappy he was, and they had heard that Driftpile had closed, but they did not know what had happened to him.[28] In December, Moore wrote to Northern Affairs giving the patient's whereabouts and confidently asserting that Sperry would relay information about the man and that this should alleviate his homesickness and the fears of his family.[29] Although one might disagree with the former assumption, at least the patient was in a place where he could get expert attention for his particular physical disability, which would have been almost impossible at Coppermine at that time. This sequence of events seems to have been fairly typical of the arbitrary "disposal" of Inuit patients, the lack of communication between the various government units involved, and the frequent disregard of the rights and wishes of the patients and their families.

In 1955 an official at Northern Affairs conducted a file study on Inuit discharged from hospital to estimate the numbers needing the still nonexistent rehabilitation services.[30] He came up with a figure of 15 per cent of TB patients and 3 per cent of general patients, but his figures were questionable and the file data inadequate to reach any valid conclusions. In any case, his study seems to have been ignored.

As the number of Inuit coming south increased, so did the appeals from the medical superintendents of the sanatoria. Dr Fiddes at Moose Factory Indian Hospital wrote in December 1955:

It seems far too severe a break to bring these people from the warmth and comfort of sanatorium life and expect them to go back and live in snow houses without any period of readaptation ... Must we hold cured patients in MFIH more or less indefinitely? Must we put these people on aircraft and send them up to the North villages regardless of the advice of the people responsible there? Is it possible for us to accommodate these people in some intermediate way by means of hostel care or boarding out care in Moose Factory ... where they would at least have housing, warmth and food?[31]

When Rudnicki drew up his five-year plan for the development of welfare services, he included plans for a proposed rehabilitation centre at Iqaluit. Construction of this centre, on the site of the present village of Apex, began in the summer of 1956. By July 1957 its first superintendent, R.J. Green, had been appointed and instructions were going out about the selection of patients and arrangements for their transfer from hospital.[32] This first rehabilitation centre finally opened in September 1957 with accommodation for 24 single people and six family units. In a 1957 letter to the secretary of the Treasury Board regarding funding, F.J.G. Cunningham described the centre as follows:

[It will house] patients who are at present boarding in hospital and are too handicapped to be discharged to their former way of life or Eskimos who have been discharged already but are not able to become self-sufficient because of their hospital experience.

The purpose of rehabilitation at the Centre will be two-fold. It will assist Eskimos ... to learn a trade or occupation consistent with their capabilities and type of disability. It will also be a means of instructing them in the handling of money, home economics, sanitation, operation of businesses, and many different skills and attributes necessary to fit into a different type of life.

The department, through its rehabilitation staff will ... also build an economic base at Iqaluit and other communities.

Eskimos will be rehabilitated in two successive stages which will be referred to as Eskimos on "Status A" and those on "Status B."

Under "Status A," residents of the Centre will be trainees in the process of acquiring many different kinds of vocational, social and economic skills. They will be dependent on the Centre for food, shelter and clothing. Under "Status B," Eskimos will have made a physical break with the Centre and will be in jobs or established in small businesses under the Eskimo Loan Fund in the community. Departmental officers will continue to provide supervision and assistance to Eskimos on "Status B" until they are thought to be self-sufficient and productive, and fully rehabilitated to a new way of life.[33]

Inuit in transit through Iqaluit, mainly between their homes and hospital, were also to be accommodated in the centre.

The centre opened without its full complement of staff, but residents and Inuit in transit were soon arriving. In August, Green outlined the projects planned for the first year: coffee shop in the centre's dining hall; bakery; bath house; weekly movies; women's workshop producing local-type clothing; carving and craftwork; organized hunts for meat and skins; men's workshop for carpentry, etc.; packaging and shipping articles for sale or display; and possibly a coffee shop at the local air base.[34] Proceeds from the projects were to go into the general funding of the centre to reduce the costs of operation. The residents, all of whom contributed to the projects or to the operation of the centre, were to be paid a weekly allowance of $2 for an adult or $1 for a child.

By January 1960, the centre had a resident population of 47 and a transient population of 16.[35] By April 1961, it consisted of 35 buildings, which were used as residences for rehabilitants and their families, transit centres for adults or children, workshops, warehouses, a kitchen, and a dining hall. Peter Murdoch, the superintendent of the centre, was assisted by a mixed staff of Inuit and whites, consisting of Abraham Okpik as program director, Elijah Menarek as

Table 20
Graduates from Rehabilitation Centre at Iqaluit, 1958–61

	1958	1959	1960	1961 to Nov.	Total
Into wage employment	2	6	3	6	17
Back to the land	1	2	1	3	7
Totals	3	8	4	9	24

Source: National Archives of Canada, RG85 (Int. 95), 1934: A252–4/169.

arts and crafts manager, four supervisors of special projects, and a clerical staff.[36]

By the beginning of the 1960s, the program had been enlarged to include some academic subjects and coaching in the basic commercial skills needed for the management of small businesses. In 1961 T.B. Golding, one of the adult education teachers from the federal school that had also been opened in Iqaluit, was seconded to the centre to run a program of specially tailored courses for individuals or small groups of trainees. These classes usually included grade-school-level courses in arithmetic, writing, English, and general knowledge in order to build on the limited schooling that most of the residents had received; plus such subjects as typing, bookkeeping, accounting, practical science, and machine shop, depending on what job the trainee was aiming for.[37]

In November 1961, NAB records showed that 24 trainees had graduated from the centre since its opening in 1957 (see table 20).[38] A further 10 were regarded as permanent residents, and a further 18 were in training. Many of these individuals were members (or, indeed, supporters) of a family that lived at the centre in "married quarters" and received rations while the trainee followed his or her program. As in the hospitals, the handicrafts program was one of the most successful at the rehabilitation centres. By 1964, the Iqaluit centre's handicraft program had developed into a sizable commercial venture with a revenue of around $40,000 annually. It had a markedly positive influence on craftspeople in the local community and surrounding settlements, for whom it provided a sales organization.[39]

The second rehabilitation centre was set up in 1961 at Inuvik, rather than at Aklavik as had been planned so long before. This centre also catered to the Indian population of the area. Projects here included log cutting, booming and saw milling, construction of log houses, fishing, food processing, chicken raising, garment manufacturing, and the operation of sales outlets. In the first year of operation 93 people earned over $50,000 through their participation in these projects.[40]

A third rehabilitation centre, called the Keewatin Re-establishment Project, ran in Rankin Inlet from 1960 to 1963; but this was as much related to the starvation and displacement of people resulting from a failure of the caribou in the Keewatin barrens as to the need to rehabilitate TB patients.[41] At first, it was run as a make-work project on the same sort of allowance system as at Iqaluit; but when Robert Williamson was made superintendent early in 1961, he changed the system to one of straight pay for quality and production, giving an allowance based on need only to those who were unable to work productively. The project was much hampered by lack of funds and shortage of staff, possibly because the federal government had decided to phase out the settlement of Rankin Inlet after 1963 when, as it had known since 1958, the nickel mine was due to close down.[42]

While the project was in operation, programs at Rankin Inlet, as at Inuvik, concentrated on the practicalities of improving living conditions in the local community and diversifying the local economy. They focused on hunting, fishing (including net making), dog raising, a bakery, a greenhouse, and stove repairing, as well as the usual lucrative handicrafts and store. When the project closed in 1963, Williamson left the Department of Northern Affairs and National Resources (NANR) but stayed on in Rankin Inlet. He remained there for the next 17 years, supporting himself by doing independent field research, writing, and hunting. Meanwhile, he devoted considerable energy to helping the local community develop into the relatively thriving administrative, communication, and cultural centre that it is today.

The rehabilitation services offered by the Iqaluit and Inuvik centres were eventually made available to all residents of the Northwest Territories, as were the other welfare services developed by the division. For the Inuit TB convalescents, they were most important in the 1960s, before the educational system had begun to catch up with the dearth of opportunities for both children and adults to learn alternate ways of livelihood to the traditional ones, and before the settlements developed into the more sophisticated hamlets that they are today.

In the 1960s the federal government moved towards establishing a quasi-provincial system of government in the Northwest Territories, though it kept the administration firmly in the hands of white civil servants. In 1959 the Arctic Division of NANR disappeared and its functions were split among three divisions (Education, Industrial, and Welfare) and the office of the administrator of the Arctic. The headquarters were all still in Ottawa, but regional offices were opened in Churchill, Iqaluit, Quebec, and the Mackenzie region.[43] In 1962 the federal vote was extended to the whole of the Northwest Territories by adding the districts of Keewatin and Franklin to the Mackenzie River riding – geographically an enormous constituency, though small in the number of voters.

In 1966 NANR was converted to the Department of Indian Affairs and Northern Development (DIAND), and the transfer of local government functions and public service from federal to territorial level proceeded apace. Only two years later the department was reorganized as its functions gradually disappeared, and by 1970 the transfer of most functions (and the public servants in the North who carried them out) to the NWT government had been completed. NWT officials assumed control over the Eastern Arctic and the islands, and federal programs for Arctic Quebec were transferred to the Indian-Eskimo Affairs program of DIAND.[44] Ottawa still remained in virtual control of the territory, however, for the legislative assembly in Yellowknife was a hybrid body, composed of some elected members and some appointees of the federal government. Not until 1979 did the federal government give the territory the right to elect all its own legislators.

Until 1988, health-care responsibility was shared between the Department of Health of the NWT government and the Medical Services branch of the federal government's Department of National Health and Welfare. The federal department gradually relinquished control over facilities and programs as regional boards of health were set up in the territory.[45] In 1987, for instance, the Medical Services branch operated a public-health program for all residents of the territory; it ran two hospitals (at Inuvik and Fort Simpson) and had 30 nursing stations, five health centres, and a number of health stations in the Mackenzie, Inuvik, and Keewatin zones. The Department of Health of the Northwest Territories was responsible for four hospitals (at Yellowknife, Hay River, Fort Smith, and Iqaluit) and had 12 nursing stations and one health centre in the Baffin region. It also managed the hospital insurance and health-care plans and legislated ordinances that controlled health activities in the territory.[46] In 1988 the remaining federal health responsibilities in the Northwest Territories were transferred to the territorial government, with the exception of noninsured health programs, which Health and Welfare continued to provide for status indians (Dene) and Inuit, and for other residents on contract.[47]

The NWT Department of Health reported in 1990: "A network of facilities now exists through which clinical services can be provided to all residents. Services are provided on an outpatient or inpatient basis, either on-site at a base hospital or health centre in the NWT, or if it is found to be medically necessary, in a facility outside the NWT ... The system ... operates on the principle of delegation of responsibility for the management and delivery of services – prevention, treatment, rehabilitation, or care to Regional Boards."[48]

Because of the great distances between many of the settlements and the few specialized medical facilities, the Department of Health subsidizes medical travel costs for people who do not have access to insured benefits through employer plans or other coverage. But as Dr Willis pointed out in 1963, there are bound to be some problems: "Because of the ... isolation of [many of its people] in small, widely dispersed groups, the people of the Northwest Territories cannot expect to enjoy a completely modern and readily available health service. There comes an end point in planning and in administration where it becomes logistically impossible and financially unreasonable to try to provide professional services at every resident's elbow. Those who insist on living in tiny groups far from lines of communication and trade centres must expect, like pioneers, to take some risks."[49]

The facilities available today are basically the same as those set up by Health and Welfare. Some patients are still sent to hospitals outside the Northwest Territories, though not necessarily for tuberculosis. Many, for example, go from the Baffin to Montreal hospitals, or from the Keewatin to Churchill, for maternity care.[50] But the percentage of funds spent on such care has dropped markedly (from 37 per cent in fiscal year 1984–85 to 21 per cent in 1989–90) as the number of hospital beds in the Northwest Territories has risen (from 410 in 1984–85 to 462 in 1988–89).[51]

None of the four little hospitals opened by the missionaries more than 60 years ago is still operating as a general hospital. Those at Aklavik closed when the federal government moved its operations in the district to a new site at Inuvik in the late 1950s and built a hospital there. St Luke's at Pangnirtung was replaced by a federal hospital at Iqaluit and a nursing station in Pangnirtung in the early 1970s. The old building, slightly enlarged, is now the Arthur Turner Training School, which trains Inuit Anglican priests for work in the Arctic. At Chesterfield Inlet, Ste-Thérèse's, which is still run by the Grey Nuns, switched in 1977 to providing highly specialized care to Inuit handicapped patients. In December 1988 there were nine severely handicapped permanent residents suffering from a variety of afflictions, brought on primarily by tuberculous meningitis, and requiring constant attention. Besides the main hospital building and staff quarters, the hospital complex now includes a greenhouse, a reservoir, an enormous larder for dry goods storage, and two oil heaters.[52]

Meningitis is no longer the scourge of young TB patients in the Arctic that it used to be, and Ste-Thérèse's may run out of patients in time. But as the NWT Department of Health has pointed out, tuberculosis as a problem will continue "as long as inadequate housing and over-crowding are common."[53] From time to time there is a flare-up in one community or another, for instance, in Repulse Bay in 1988–89. In those two years the number of cases among Inuit of the Northwest Territories rose to 55 from a total of 35 for 1986–87.[54] However, the importance of TB in the community at large is now outweighed by the extremely high suicide and infant-death rates – both of which are more than twice the Canadian rate – and by a growing concern over AIDS.

CHAPTER ELEVEN

Distinct but Similar:

The Epidemic in Quebec and Newfoundland

QUEBEC

In the 1950s some 2,000 Inuit were living along the coast of the Ungava Peninsula in northern Quebec, as they had for thousands of years. The Hudson's Bay Company (HBC) had set up trading posts in Rupert's Land around James Bay in the seventeenth century and had expanded into Inuit territory by opening a post at what is now Umiujaq in 1749. Other posts followed during the nineteenth and early twentieth centuries, until by 1930 there were trading posts dotted around the coast at most of what are now the Inuit villages of northern Quebec. After the traders came the missionaries, notably the Moravians, who extended their chain of missions in Labrador along the coast to Kuujjuak in 1825. Kuujjuak was also the site of the first Roman Catholic mission in the area in 1871 and of an Anglican mission in 1900. Both these churches gradually extended their missions to cover most of the trading posts around the Ungava and Hudson Bay coasts.

In 1912 the whole territory was designated by the Canadian government as part of the Province of Quebec, but the federal government continued to treat it in the main as though it were part of the Northwest Territories. The coastal settlements were included on the Eastern Arctic Patrol run, meteorological stations were set up at various points, RCMP posts were established, fur taxes collected, and so on. As in the Baffin, what services were available to the people (except from those on the Eastern Arctic Patrol) were provided by the missions and the traders. Apart from accepting the provincial fur tax, the province took virtually no interest in the area.[1]

Both levels of government, in fact, seemed only too anxious to leave the area to the people, the traders, and the missionaries. It was

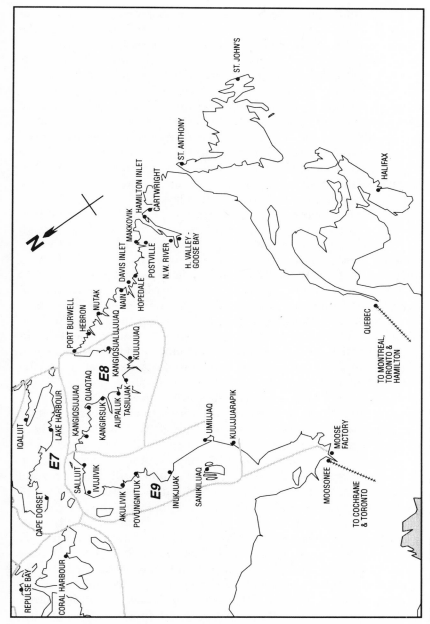

Map 3   Inuit Villages in Quebec and Labrador (N.F. Fielding, Thames Label & Litho)

the actions of the HBC which first forced a greater measure of involvement onto the federal government. The Great Depression of the 1930s, with its severe drop in fur prices, hit the Inuit of this area particularly hard, and the HBC advanced survival credits to them. The HBC then billed the federal government, which promptly passed the bill on to the provincial government. The Quebec government, however, refused to pay, maintaining that the Inuit were a federal responsibility, and the matter went to the Supreme Court of Canada. In 1939 the Supreme Court ruled in favour of Quebec's position. Thereafter, the federal government was free – indeed, obliged – to provide necessary services to the Inuit of northern Quebec (and, by extension, the Inuit of the rest of Canada) and to govern them directly; at least, according to Canadian law.

The actual situation of the Inuit, of course, did not materially change. They continued to be administered from Ottawa through the war years and the 1950s, and to be included in whatever provisions for relief, family allowances, and other measures the federal government made. When Health and Welfare took over responsibility for Inuit health services in 1945, the Ungava Inuit were included in the program of nursing stations, surveys, and southern hospitalization, with all its traumas and successes, just like their people farther north. Federal schools were opened in some settlements and taught only in English, and government personnel generally operated in English. Although this caused extra problems for local Inuit who were sent out to hospital (because they were generally sent to French-speaking Quebec hospitals), the same problems were experienced by the many Inuit from other areas who were sent to Quebec hospitals.

In 1962, however, René Lévesque, who at the time was Quebec's minister of natural resources, visited the area. He was shocked by the anglicization of the Inuit and by the lack of Quebec presence in a part of the province that he recognized as potentially rich in natural resources – and particularly ripe for hydro development.[2] This led to the formation in 1963 of the Direction générale du Nouveau-Québec (in Lévesque's ministry), which was to be responsible for all Quebec government action in northern Quebec, except in the areas of justice, and lands and forests. Discussions between the federal and Quebec governments also took place that year, and they eventually led to an agreement stipulating that Quebec would gradually take over the administration of the area, beginning with education and health – really to absorb it, and its people, into the province. The Quebec government built nursing stations in settlements still lacking them, and it installed a parallel school system. In the Quebec government schools, classes were taught in Inuktitut for the first three years and in French thereafter.

Through the sixties and seventies the two levels of government operated in the area in parallel. The federal government built housing, developed Inuit cooperatives, and continued to run the medical service and nursing stations that it had established there. The provincial government concentrated on schools and technical and engineering projects, and started nursing centres in communities that had not yet been provided with them by Health and Welfare. In 1967 a small provincial hospital was opened at Kuujjuak and provided a dental clinic, an x-ray department, visiting physicians for Ungava Bay villages, and referrals to Quebec hospitals for specialist treatment. By 1969 the federal government had ceded medical services in the Ungava Bay area to the province, but it still maintained services along the Hudson Bay coast.

The James Bay hydroelectric project dominated the early 1970s. Signature of the accord in 1975, with the bulk of the Inuit communities represented by the Northern Quebec Inuit Association (now Makivik), led to a hastening of the federal government's retreat in the face of the formation of local (Kativik) educational and health boards. Three Inuit villages – Povungnituk, Ivujivik, and part of Salluit – did not sign the accord and formed a dissident organization, the Inuit Tungavingat Nunamini; this led to a reduction in many services in these communities ("au prix d'une diminution dans bien des services," to quote from a Government of Quebec publication)[3] and more administrative difficulties for the government departments involved. Special agreements have since been worked out between the two opposing Inuit factions – for instance, as regards schools and health services. But the disagreement still stands, and patients from Povungnituk may be sent to hospital in Iqaluit rather than to a hospital in Quebec.

Over the years, the Montreal General Hospital and the Centre hospitalier de l'Université Laval (CHUL) have specialized in the care of the Inuit, the latter receiving most of the patients who have been sent south by the medical authorities at Kuujjuak for specialist treatment since the centre was established. In 1978 CHUL was chosen by the Kativik Health Board to oversee the medical services in northern Quebec, including specialist availability, staff recruitment and training, and public health. A special section, Projet Nord, was set up to do this.

In 1980 the federal government withdrew completely from the health care of the Inuit in northern Quebec, and the clinics and nursing centres along the coast came under the control of the main Ungava medical centre at Kuujjuaq, except for the dissident villages where the facilities are run directly by CHUL. In 1982 a new and larger regional hospital for the Ungava was opened at Kuujjuak, providing a wide range of out-patient and in-patient care, and in 1986 a similar regional centre (Innuulisivik) was opened at Povung-nituk for the Hudson Bay coast. The villages are now organized as municipal corporations, as they are in the Northwest Territories, with mayors and elected councillors, and (with the exception of the dis-sident villages) they are represented on fhe Kativik regional council, which plays an important administrative role in the areas of health, social services, the environment, education, and economic develop-ment. But the final decisions and financial resources (except for the money from the James Bay 1 agreement, which is administered by Makivik) are still in the hands of the various Quebec ministries that have interests in the North.

As far as tuberculosis is concerned, the same general trends are apparent as among other Inuit, except for two things. First, the number of new active cases reported in the late 1960s in the northern Quebec villages suggests a lower incidence rate than in the rest of the Inuit population of Canada (see table 21).[4] Second, the incidence was generally higher through the 1970s than in the rest of the Inuit community, and although it was steadily declining, it was dropping only half as quickly as in the Northwest Territories.

There may be several factors contributing to these discrepancies. For a start, medical coverage of the area may have suffered in the 1960s during the arguments about jurisdiction and the switchover of responsibility between the two senior levels of government. For example, the federal government began winding down some of its services (such as the Eastern Arctic Patrol ship, which stopped calling at Quebec posts some years before it was withdrawn altogether) before the provincial government had its own organization well in place. Secondly, in the 1970s when there was increased diagnostic activity in the area, medical practice was provided mainly by young, inexperienced doctors who had rarely, if ever, seen a case of tuber-culosis down south. Although they were conditioned to expect TB among the Inuit, they may not clearly have distinguished the syn-drome and usually left the area before they had time to become experienced.[5] Dr Turcotte, an epidemiologist with Projet Nord at CHUL, suggested that there had been an added complication for inexperienced physicians, namely, the previous overadministration of BCG vaccinations (some people had received as many as 16).[6] He

Table 21
Tuberculosis Morbidity among Quebec Inuit, 1966–90, Compared with All Inuit
in Canada (Rates per 100,000 Population)

| | Number of cases in Quebec | | | Rates: 5-year averages[1] | | | |
| | | | | Total cases | | New active cases only | |
Year	New active	Reactivated	Total	Quebec	Canada	Quebec	Canada
1966	25	1	26				
1967	9	2	11				
1968	8	0	8				
1969	11	0	11				
1970	24	3	27	449	1,325	416	1,085
1971	–	–	56				
1972	–	–	11				
1973	32	5	37				
1974	8	0	8				
1975	11	2	13	652	391	439[2]	303
1976	7	1	8				
1977	11	6	17				
1978	16	5	21				
1979	4	1	5				
1980	10	1	11	255	149	212	113
1981	8	2	10				
1982	13	3	16				
1983	29	1	30				
1984	3	1	4				
1985	14	1	15	296	126	264	96
1986	9	0	9				
1987	7	0	7				
1988	3	0	3				
1989	1	0	1				
1990	3	0	3	79	84	79	66

Sources: Quebec data for 1966–70 and all Canadian data are from Statistics Canada, tuberculosis
statistics, morbidity and mortality, cats. 83-206 and 82-212, and health reports, cat. 82-003s10.
Quebec data for 1971–90 are from Ministère de la Santé et des Services sociaux (MSSS),
Government of Quebec, annual report, 1991.
[1] Averages calculated by the author, using Statistics Canada's Inuit population figures for all
Canada; an estimated Quebec Inuit population figure of 3,700 for Quebec data, 1966–70; and MSSS
figures for Quebec data, 1971–90.
[2] Three-year average.

suggested that the 1970s data may reflect "false" diagnoses based on positive Mantoux tests found in such people, who had not actually developed tuberculosis. Thus, there emerged in the 1970s a discrepancy between the number of cases reported in the statistics and the number of tuberculous patients who could be observed "on the ground" by a visiting experienced physician.

It seems likely, therefore, that the 1960s figures underestimate the incidence in the area and that the 1970s figures are an overestimate. Figures for the 1980s, particularly the later years, suggest that the Quebec program is now working fairly effectively. Dr Beauchesne, who is in charge of tuberculosis control in Quebec at the Ministère de la Santé et des Services sociaux (Department of Health and Social Services) maintains that there was no particular reason for the unusually high incidence in 1983. He thinks the explanation is simply that some hunting families were missed on surveys the previous year and that the disease was therefore transmitted to other members of the group before the patient could be diagnosed and isolated.[7]

Since the Quebec government entered the field of health care for the Inuit of the Ungava and Hudson Bay coasts, it seems to have successfully established hospital treatment in the North and to be working to train local people to staff the northern medical services so that a greater degree of stability, continuity, and experience can be achieved.

NEWFOUNDLAND

The smallest group of Inuit in Canada are those of Newfoundland, who numbered less than 1,000 in the 1950s. They live along the northern part of the coast of Labrador which, intermittently, has been visited by Europeans since the eleventh century, when the Vikings established their colony of Vinland at L'Anse aux Meadows at the tip of the northern peninsula of Newfoundland. Many traces of stone houses and stone-protected tombs, such as the Norsemen built, have been found in the area.

In their Vinland voyages from Greenland, the Vikings met and fought with the Inuit, though at that time there were no Inuit living near their colonies in Greenland. In the fourteenth century, the Inuit moved south down the west coast of Greenland, and there was more contact between the two groups. About this time the climate deteriorated rapidly. Contact between Europe and the Viking colonies was lost, and when Europeans again visited the area in the sixteenth century, the Inuit were in complete possession. A few ruins were all that remained of the Viking settlements. It is not clear whether the deterioration in the weather, attacks from the Inuit, disease, or a combination of all these factors caused the collapse of what had been quite well-established colonies. Since the Scandinavian countries had much tuberculosis at the time and since evidence of spinal TB has been found in the Viking graveyards, tuberculosis has been suggested as a contributory factor.

In the sixteenth century, fishermen from Portugal, France, and England began to use the fishing grounds off Labrador and to interact with the Inuit living and fishing along the coast. Explorers from the same countries used the waters and occasionally landed on their way to the Gulf of St Lawrence or Hudson Bay. In the mid-eighteenth century, the Moravian church from Bavaria, which by then was well established in Greenland, began to set up missions in northern Labrador, and from then on it played somewhat the same role for the Inuit communities there as the Oblates and the Anglicans played in the Arctic. The first missions were at Nain and Makkovik; later ones at Hebron and Hopedale. Although their settlers rarely included doctors and they set up no hospitals, the Moravians brought some practical nursing and education to the people as well as their particular brand of Christianity, and they tried to broaden the people's economic base.

The Moravians kept very good records of all deaths, and from these it appears that death from pulmonary tuberculosis was a frequent occurrence; but the arrival of the missionaries and the HBC traders, and a few fishing families from southern Newfoundland who soon followed them, did not cause a mass outbreak of the disease. This seems to be a further indication that tuberculosis had been present in the communities for a long time, probably brought by the Vikings, so that some natural resistance to the disease had been built up in the people. For the next two centuries, tuberculosis remained a troublesome disease, occasionally reaching epidemic proportions in the wake of outbreaks of other infections, such as measles, influenza, or whooping cough.

The first medical services came to Labrador through Wilfred Grenfell, who heard of the plight of the Grand Banks fishing families when he was a young doctor working for the National Mission to Deep Sea Fishermen in the North Sea. In 1892 the mission sent him to Newfoundland on an exploratory trip, and by August he was off the southern Labrador coast greeting an "incredulous people, an almost-forgotten race who didn't know what a 'real' doctor was."[8] Grenfell went as far north as Hopedale, covering in two months some 1,800 kilometres of uncharted coast and treating 900 sick and injured people among the fishermen and their families. He found whole

families riddled with tuberculosis, and also found rampant malnutrition, scurvy, beri-beri, and rickets. Apart from the Inuit, who were
mainly on the northern section of the coast, and a few Indians who
came from inland to trade at the HBC post at Davis Inlet, the people
were summer fishing families on schooners from Newfoundland or
year-round "liveyers" living in inadequate shacks, exploited by the
fish buyers, and surviving mainly on potatoes, flour, molasses, and
a few fish. They had no services of any sort available to them and
were in too severe straits to help themselves.

Back in St John's, Grenfell energetically pressed the authorities to
provide some medical services. That winter, he began the fundraising and lobbying activities that eventually resulted in the Grenfell
Mission and, in 1912, the formation of the International Grenfell
Association. Long before that, however, Grenfell had organized the
medical services on the coast, expanding them as he acquired the
money or the personnel to run them – and often before there was a
sufficiency of either. Apart from showing goodwill and giving permission for Grenfell to go ahead with the good work, the Newfoundland authorities seem to have been content to leave it all in his hands,
having their own full with the needs of the island itself and their
chronic lack of money.

In 1893, Grenfell opened a hospital at Battle Harbour, and a motor
launch was donated for visiting the coastal settlements. Next year, a
summer-only hospital was opened at Indian Harbour farther north,
and in 1895 a small hospital boat was provided. Grenfell travelled
extensively each winter across the United States and Canada as well
as Britain, raising money for the work and persuading many excellent
medical specialists to spend a few months or a year working in
Labrador alongside the very few permanent staff of the mission. In
1901 the hospital at St Anthony on the northern tip of the island of
Newfoundland was opened, and in the following two years exten-
sions were made to the hospitals at Battle Harbour and Indian Harbour. Another small hospital was set up at North West River in 1915.

Grenfell had been impressed by the efforts of the Moravian
Brothers among the Inuit in northern Labrador, and through his
mission he tried various ways to help the more southerly Labrador
population to improve their economic status and living conditions.
In association with his hospitals, he set up workshops, handicraft
centres, greenhouses, dry docks, farms, cooperative stores, travelling
libraries, orphanages, and even, for a short time, a reindeer herd.
During the 1920s and 1930s, several nursing stations and schools
were opened; three more small hospitals were built, a 30-bed TB

annex was opened at St Anthony, and radio stations were set up at St Anthony and North West River.

But these efforts in preventive medicine, and the hospital facilities of the mission, were available mainly to the predominantly white fishing communities of southern Labrador and northern Newfoundland. The Inuit lived on the coast northward from the Hamilton Inlet–Goose Bay area to Hebron, and here the medical services were more restricted, despite the cooperation of the Moravian Brothers, the HBC traders, and the occasional visiting doctor. Before World War II, the closest x-ray machine was at Cartwright, too far south to be of help to the people of northern Labrador. The rather grim situation is described by Dr W.A. Paddon, who spent his childhood in the area and eventually took over the hospital at North West River, which had been established at the beginning of World War I by his father, Dr H. Paddon:

Until the end of the Second World War ... the total resources of the area consisted of a ten bed hospital at North West River, and the care of the outlying settlements was restricted to a patrol of the coast by summer in the small hospital boat "Maraval" and a visit to parts of it by dog-team in the winter. The territory, even using modern air transport, is over four hundred miles long, and over eight hundred as the dog-team travels. During the war there was no resident medical officer available for the North West River hospital, and this station was operated as a dispensary and nursing establishment.[9]

At the same time, the old social economic patterns of life had been changing, and by the end of World War II the situation was parlous indeed. The international markets for fur and salt fish, the main products of Labrador, had declined, adding to the already severe hardship in the area. A large air base had been established at Goose Bay, and like the bases in the Arctic, it brought both the chance of employment for migrants from the northern villages and epidemics of acute infectious diseases, which were then carried back to the villages and spread along the coast. The migrants, who generally lived in "a sprawling shanty town on the outskirts of the military area ... known as Happy Valley or Hamilton Valley ... presented an especially difficult problem in tuberculosis control."[10]

Owing to the sporadic nature of the medical attention available to the people in the northern villages, tuberculosis had previously been treated mainly indirectly, through attempts to develop the economy and improve the living conditions and hygiene of the people, and by evacuating a few of the most severely sick to the hospitals farther south. But the poverty in the area, the overcrowding for warmth in the severe winters, the increasing epidemics of other infections (which led to fresh waves of tuberculosis cases), and the people's unwillingness to go to hospital for fear of dying away from their family, resulted in an alarming increase in tuberculosis during the war. Paddon estimated that the mortality rate for TB in the area was more than 400 per 100,000 population and that for the Inuit communities it was much higher, perhaps exceeding 900 per 100,000.[11]

The doctor who visited the villages two or three times a year, by boat in the summer or by dog team in the winter, spent most of his time on emergency minor surgery, extracting teeth, and fitting eyeglasses that were urgently needed by "women who could no longer see to do the fine stitching of sealskin boots and clothing for their families ... The only patients who were likely to get the hospital treatment they needed were those who were lucky enough to be sick on one of the rare occasions when transportation was available for them – and too sick to say no."[12]

These hard and frustrating dogsled patrols by the doctors were, however, to produce a dividend that was built on to make the TB control system developed after the war more effective. It was the same dividend that had been built up in the Arctic by people such as Dr Schaefer or the nurses in the scattered nursing stations (but had generally been ignored by the southern-based *C.D. Howe* patrol, with unhappy results). As Dr Paddon put it, "These preparatory years were ... to provide invaluable experience and a closeness of touch with the people which could have been achieved in no other way. Medical personnel sharing the homes and the bread of these people, as well as the hard physical labour and sometimes downright hardship of dog-team travel, quickly achieved their respect. The confidence thus won was to prove most valuable in carrying out the much more effectual medical programs of the next few years."[13]

With the end of the war and the return of physicians such as Paddon from the forces, it became possible for the Grenfell Mission to make an energetic new approach to the medical problems of the area and, in particular, to develop an effective program to control tuberculosis. The first step was to x-ray as many people as possible. To this end an x-ray machine was installed at North West River in 1947, and a second one was installed in 1948 on the small hospital ship *Maraval*, which visited the coastal settlements each summer. The films were taken at each stop, generally on the northward trip, and were developed on board so that patients' counselling, retakes, and evacuation for treatment could be done on the way south.

Considerable thought was given to the question of the selection of patients for hospital treatment and to the general presentation of the survey and treatment program in the north shore communities. As Paddon explained, it was "clearly understood that all who came south came freely of their own accord, and that anyone could leave hospital and return if travelling conditions permitted." Patients were also assured that they would not be put in a ward where no one else could speak their language, though this proved rather difficult to achieve within the usual hospital administrative rules.

It was decided to reserve the few available beds for two categories of patients: the young, clearly sick, but not too far advanced cases, who had a good chance of a relatively speedy recovery; and people who were clearly a public-health menace in terms of spreading the disease (usually, chronic, far-advanced cases, who were living in close proximity to their families). These criteria were chosen partly as a way of using the available resources to greatest effect, either in curing patients or in preventing the spread of disease; and partly as a way of trying to overcome the communities' resistance to evacuation by balancing the likely deaths in hospital of patients whose TB was far advanced with the likelihood of cure for the younger group.

The difference between the approach and operation of the Grenfell Association's TB program in Newfoundland and that mounted by Health and Welfare in the Eastern Arctic stands out in Paddon's account. In 1948, the first year that the x-ray survey was done, 329 people were seen. Of these, 48 (or 14.6 per cent) were considered active (and a further 10.6 per cent considered suspicious), of whom more than 30 agreed to go south for treatment. This led to great difficulties with transportation. The coastal steamships, which had no facilities for isolation and had a natural fear of the disease, refused to carry tuberculous passengers, and the *Maraval* officially had berths for only two. Since the *Maraval*'s annual visit to the settlements was the only means of getting the TB patients out, the ship and her crew accepted the risks of the additional passengers. Beds were made up directly on the deck, in the dispensary, and elsewhere, and the ship, both that year and on several occasions in the next few years, carried more than 30 patients south, fortunately with no mishaps. As Paddon put it, "It was morally impossible to leave many people behind in the knowledge that to do so might cost them their lives".[14] Known or suspected cases remaining at home were followed up to some extent during the winter by a combined dog-team and aerial patrol.

The next year, only 250 x-rays were taken because the ship was too busy with routine clinic and dispensary work, but the results showed some improvement, the percentage of active or suspicious cases having dropped from 25.2 per cent in 1948 to 17.6 per cent in 1949. After the first year's experience, the doctors were more confident of their x-ray interpretation, and plates that had previously been considered suspicious were now firmly interpreted as positive. But the evacuation of so many active cases the previous year had had some effect, and the number of far-advanced open lesions was reduced. The safe return of several minimal cases who had been evacuated the previous season, and letters from friends and relations who had spent the winter in hospital, encouraged others (even the gravely ill who had refused to go out before) now to accept hospital treatment for themselves.

The hospital treatment, particularly for the more serious cases, had also shifted from the techniques of the 1930s and 1940s in a way that was less threatening to the Inuit. All the surgical cases were sent to St Anthony, where thoracoplasty had been the favoured procedure. While it was a very effective curative treatment, this mutilating operation was dreaded by Inuit and Indian hunters, who were dependent on their physical fitness for their livelihood. When, in the late 1940s, streptomycin became available and was increasingly used, Dr G.W. Thomas, the surgeon then in charge at St Anthony's, began to use segmental resection, or lobectomy, as the surgical treatment of choice. Dr Paddon wrote in 1957, "The results have been highly gratifying, and the Eskimo and Indian patients in particular have lost much of their dread of the possible consequences of going away to hospital. The idea of resecting a lesion is one which an Eskimo can appreciate, for in his own folklore illness is almost always caused by something broken which must be repaired or something bad which must be removed."[15]

Meanwhile, the community leaders and the government both helped foster the TB program as far as they could. The Newfoundland Department of Welfare introduced fuel and cash allowances for families when the breadwinner went into hospital; and if both parents were hospitalized, arrangements were made for their children to go to boarding school, preferably near the hospital to which their parents had been admitted. The village elders supported the program, and attempts were made to improve housing for the returning patients; and the Moravian Mission at Nain broadcast news about the progress of patients in hospital, as well as broadcasting talks on TB in Inuktitut and English.

Another important event happened in Newfoundland in 1949: it joined the Canadian confederation. As an immediate consequence of this, family allowances, old-age pensions, widows' allowances, and disability pensions brought new cash to the chronically hard-up

Newfoundland and Labrador society, leading to better food and clothes and improvements in housing.[16] No special status for Indians and Inuit was included in the terms of union between Newfoundland and Canada, and there has been an ongoing debate over which level of government is actually responsible for providing Newfoundland natives with the services that are provided for other natives in Canada by the federal government and for non-natives by the various provincial governments. However, the Indian Health Service of the federal Department of National Health and Welfare began subsidizing the hospital treatment of tuberculous native patients at a daily rate of $22 per patient, and during the 1950s and 1960s it paid for the building of four new nursing stations for the Grenfell Association at Nain, Davis Inlet, Makkovik, and Hopedale.[17]

This was the first substantial support the Grenfell Association had ever received from government. Even so, 60 per cent of its funds came from donations, which were raised mainly in the United States. For a long time, both the provincial and federal governments were content to leave the medical, educational, and social services for the Northern Peninsula and Labrador in the hands of the Moravian Brothers and the Grenfell Association, both of which were essentially privately funded, foreign-based institutions.

The Grenfell Association, now with a more secure and rising income, continued with its TB control program. Each summer another survey was carried out, sometimes by the association's *Maraval* and sometimes by a ship from another organization. In 1951 the Newfoundland Tuberculosis Association conducted the survey from its ship, the *Christmas Seal*, covering the coast as far as Nain; ice conditions prevented it from going on to Nutak and Hebron. In 1952–53 only follow-up work and some air evacuations were done; this was made possible by the fact that the cost was carried by the provincial government. In 1954 the federal government's Indian Health Service sponsored an x-ray and general health survey via the RCMP cutter *McBrien*. By that time, the Grenfell Association had acquired two planes through the provincial Department of Health, one stationed at St Anthony, the other at North West River, and this made its response to emergency situations very much more efficient. A new sanatorium had been built at St Anthony, and all the hospitals were filled to capacity, with more than 100 tubercular patients under treatment.

In 1955 the *Maraval* crew conducted the survey, and in 1956 the *Christmas Seal* took over again. The year 1955 was notable as the first year when not one Inuk or Indian refused to go out for hospital care. The results of the 1956 survey confirmed those of the previous two

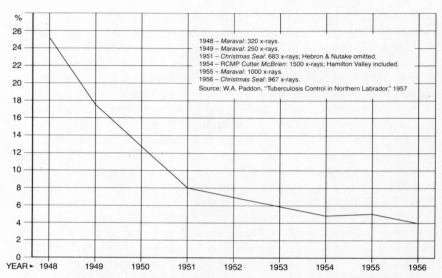

1948 – *Maraval*: 320 x-rays.
1949 – *Maraval*: 250 x-rays.
1951 – *Christmas Seal*: 683 x-rays; Hebron & Nutake omitted.
1954 – RCMP Cutter *McBrien*: 1500 x-rays; Hamilton Valley included.
1955 – *Maraval*: 1000 x-rays.
1956 – *Christmas Seal*: 967 x-rays.
Source: W.A. Paddon, "Tuberculosis Control in Northern Labrador," 1957

Figure 2   Percentage of X-ray Films Read as Active or Probably Active Tuberculosis on Summer Surveys in Labrador

years: both the proportion and the severity of cases of active tuberculosis remaining in the area were considerably lower than when the surveys had begun. The progression is shown in figure 2.

These figures relate to the entire population of the area. The Grenfell Association made no distinction between native and non-native residents – and, indeed, there was much intermarriage in the area – and Statistics Canada did not record TB data by province and origin before 1966. In 1957 there were approximately 1,500 people who were predominantly Inuit, living on the northern Labrador coast, 2,500 of white or mixed descent in the Goose Bay area, and 300 Indians in the Davis Inlet area. The most northerly communities were almost entirely Inuit.[18] Origin was, however, noted on the death of a patient. Figure 3 shows the mortality rates for the total north Labrador population and for the Inuit population from 1943 to 1956. The same dramatic fall is apparent as in the survey figures, particularly for the Inuit population. Of course, with more patients in hospital for treatment each year, the number of positive x-rays found in the community surveys was bound to fall to some extent, even without a real drop in the incidence, until the numbers of hospital patients stabilized. But this would not apply to the mortality rate. Both the incidence and the mortality rates, however, might be expected to fall gradually as, through exposure and vaccination, the population

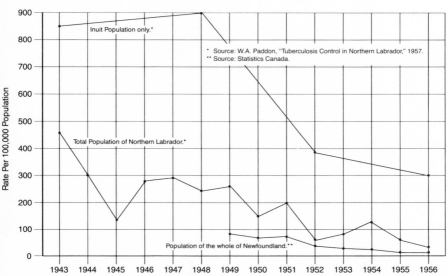

Figure 3   Tuberculosis Mortality Rates (per 100,000) for Northern Labrador, 1943–56

developed more resistance to the viral infections that in the past had been followed by outbreaks of tuberculosis in the villages affected.

Tuberculin testing and BCG vaccination of children under the age of eight were introduced in the summer of 1956 with the help of the Newfoundland Tuberculosis Association and the Department of Health, using both the *Christmas Seal* and the Beaver aircraft. There was a high proportion (74 per cent) of tuberculin negative results, as can be seen from the figures: total tuberculin tests performed, 1,293; total BCG vaccinations, 963. The percentage of children needing vaccination varied inversely with the distance from North West River hospital (see table 22). This was perhaps a reflection of the worsening economic problems as well as the greater difficulty of getting medical care in the remoter communities.[19]

The generally low proportion of positive results may be partly due to the large number of families in Hamilton Valley who had recently moved there from other parts of Canada, where tuberculosis was practically wiped out. But it may also have been a result of removing known spreaders of the disease for several years. It certainly indicated a marked improvement in a population which only 13 years before had had a death rate of over 400 per 100,000.

Public-health education in the 1950s remained at the personal doctor-individual family level, with only the most basic measures suggested (for instance, that one should provide separate dishes and

Table 22
Percentage of Children Needing Vaccination in Labrador, 1956

Town	% given BCG	Kilometres from North West River
Hamilton Valley	90	32
Postville	81	177
Hopedale	75	212
Davis Inlet	58	281
Nain	47	386
Hebron	32	547

Source: W.A. Paddon, "Tuberculosis Control in Northern Labrador" (DPH thesis, School of Hygiene and Tropical Medicine, London, 1957).

sleeping space for a sick person and that the sick should avoid coughing in the faces of others). It was thought that anything more would be counterproductive. The schools provided instruction in basic hygiene, and this sometimes spread to the parents also. The Grenfell Association ran boarding schools in southern Labrador and northern Newfoundland, and convalescent children were moved from hospital to a nearby school (even while they were still on anti-TB drugs) to complete their cure and gain strength. The schools also accepted some children from the North whose families had problems, such as both parents being in hospital, so that the children were often able to get a better education than would have been possible if they had stayed at home. The Moravian Brothers ran schools in the villages, but there the children often did not attend.[20] Drug therapy was continued for long periods after the patient's return home. It was given by a nurse, if there was a nursing station in the village, or by a designated lay worker who had been trained to administer medication. The Moravian missions again played an important part here.

During the 1960s and 1970s, the Grenfell Association maintained its TB control program of x-ray surveys, BCG vaccination, hospitalization, and examination of TB contacts in the northern Labrador communities, but it gradually scaled down its other activities as the Newfoundland government took on more responsibility for social services in the area. In the late 1950s, several Moravian missions in the Far North and their attendant villages, including Hebron, were closed by the government to save money, and the population of Nain grew accordingly.[21] Evacuations and surveys by the Christmas Seal stopped in the mid-1970s as the use of aircraft became more common and x-rays could be carried out at the new nursing stations. All women giving birth in hospital were routinely x-rayed. BCG vaccination of newborns was discontinued in 1979, after various international studies questioned its efficacy. Periodic Mantoux skin testing, followed by chemoprophylaxis if necessary, was introduced instead, starting at the pre-school level.[22]

In 1981 the Grenfell Association became the Grenfell Regional Health Services, with representatives from across the region on its board of directors, and this is the body that now provides health facilities, personnel, and services for the region. Meanwhile, the Labrador Inuit Association (LIA), which was formed in 1973, has been supplementing the efforts of the Grenfell Association and its successor by direct negotiations with the federal government for programs that are available to other Inuit groups. In the health field, the LIA is particularly concerned about the relationship between health and the social, environmental, and economic conditions in a community – a vital relationship in the control of tuberculosis.[23] The LIA is also concerned with the need to coordinate all community services and with the importance of health education and community involvement. Since 1989, through its subsidiary, the Labrador Inuit Health Commission, the LIA has operated the Non-Insured Health Benefits Program.

Throughout this period, the incidence of tuberculosis in the Labrador Inuit was gradually dropping. Statistics Canada data show that in the late 1960s there were on average still 20 times more new cases of TB among Inuit from Newfoundland than might have been expected from their proportion of the population, but this compares favourably with the factor of 30 for Canada as a whole.[24] By the late 1970s, the corresponding figures (for new and reactivated cases) had dropped to six times the expected percentage in Newfoundland and nine times the percentage in Canada as a whole. Tables 23 and 24 give the incidence as reported to Statistics Canada during the 1960s and 1970s. They show that, apart from a jump in new cases in 1969–70, the rate of new and reactivated cases declined to slightly below the rate for Inuit in the country as a whole.

In 1985 the Grenfell Regional Health Services reviewed all TB cases in northern Labrador over the period 1979–84 in order to identify high-risk groups, to establish the most effective methods of detecting cases, and to check the usefulness of the skin-testing program that had replaced the BCG vaccination program. Their findings were as follows.

- 74 per cent of TB patients were 34 or younger, 50 per cent of them being younger than 15.

Table 23
Tuberculosis Morbidity among Labrador Inuit, 1961–65, Compared with All Inuit in
Canada (Rates per 100,000 Population; Labrador Inuit Population Estimate, 1,500)

| | Numbers: Newfoundland, hospital admissions | | | Rates: 5-year averages[1] | | | |
| | | | | Total admissions | | Incidence: first admissions only | |
Year	First admissions	Readmissions	Total	Nfld	Canada	Nfld	Canada
1961	22	4	26				
1962	14	4	18				
1963	6	4	10				
1964	9	4	13				
1965	14	2	16	1,107	1,950	867	1,332

Sources: Statistics Canada, tuberculosis statistics, morbidity and mortality, cat. 83-206.
[1] Rates and averages calculated by author.

- There was considerable variation in the incidence of TB between different communities, 85 per cent of the cases coming from only three of the nine communities covered (Davis Inlet, Nain, and Sheshatshiu).
- The Innu (Indian) population was most at risk. The annual rate of new and reactivated cases per 100,000 population by ethnic groups for 1980–84 was as follows: Innu, 27 cases in a population of 740, with an average annual rate of 729.7; Inuit, 15 cases in a population of 2,204, with an average annual rate of 136.1; others, 4 cases in a population of 7,716, with an average annual rate of 10.36.
- 2.3 per cent of the surviving children born during the six years without BCG vaccination were tuberculin positive; 99 per cent of eligible children had been tested.
- 92 per cent of the cases were detected by tracing patient contacts or by consultation as a result of symptoms. Only 4 per cent were detected through routine x-rays.
- There were no deaths due to tuberculosis during the period.
- When the communities of North West River and Happy Valley, Goose Bay, and Mudlake (where the majority of the population was in the "others" category) were omitted from the calculations, the trends generally became more pronounced. For example, in 1979–84, 80 per cent of cases were 34 years or younger, and the three communities of Davis Inlet, Nain, and Sheshatshiu accounted for 93 per cent of all cases.[25]

As a result of their findings, the authors of the study suggested that routine x-rays and surveys might be discontinued in favour of

Table 24

Tuberculosis Morbidity among Labrador Inuit, 1966–85, Compared with All Inuit in Canada (Rates per 100,000 Population; Labrador Inuit Population Estimate 1,500)

| | Numbers: Newfoundland, reported cases | | | Rates: 5-year averages[1] | | | |
| | | | | Total cases | | Incidence: new active cases | |
Year	New active	Reactivated	Total	Nfld	Canada	Nfld	Canada
1966	7	2	9				
1967	8	0	8				
1968	10	0	10				
1969	17	0	17				
1970	28	4	32	1,013	1,325	933	1,085
1971	12	3	15				
1972	7	5	12				
1973	3	2	5				
1974	4	1	5				
1975	3	4	7	587	391	387	303
1976	1	0	1				
1977	2	0	2				
1978	0	1	1				
1979	–	–	1				
1980	–	–	0	67	149	67[2]	113
1981	–	–	3				
1982	–	–	7				
1983	–	–	3				
1984	–	–	2				
1985	–	–	4	253	126	–	96

Sources: Statistics Canada, tuberculosis statistics, morbidity and mortality, cats. 83-206 and 82-212, and health reports, cat. 82-003s10.

[1] Rates and averages calculated by author.

[2] Three-year average. Statistics Canada did not report new and reactivated cases separately by origin and province after 1978.

concentration on careful contact tracing and a high index of clinical suspicion of presenting symptoms; that BCGs should not be reintroduced; that communities with a low or zero incidence could be omitted from the tuberculin testing program; and that special attention should be paid to Davis Inlet (a predominantly Innu settlement like Sheshatshiu) and to any Innu patient coming for clinical consultation. They concluded that the high rate of new and reactivated cases in the region would not be lowered until the living standards of the residents improved. Their recommendations were implemented, and by 1991 the testing program was being further reduced in communities with very low rates. Careful contact tracing and suspicion of clinical symptoms remain the main emphasis of the program.[26]

The rate of infection and reinfection for the small group of Innu covered in the 1985 study seems to be higher than for any other native group in Canada at the time.[27] The rate for Labrador Inuit was only a little above the average rate for Canadian Inuit as a whole (122 per 100,000 in 1980–84) and rather better than for Inuit in Quebec during the same period (291 per 100,000).[28] It appears also that Inuit on the Labrador coast experienced the same increase in tuberculosis in 1969–71 as their neighbours along the Ungava and Hudson Bay coasts (see tables 21, 23, and 24). No explanation for this has been forthcoming from the departments of health concerned. At all events, the disease seems now to be as well under control in Labrador as anywhere in the Inuit community, and the Labrador Inuit Association seems to be taking an active part in health services for its community.

PART THREE

Conclusions

CHAPTER TWELVE

The Balance Sheet:

One Person's Point of View

So the epidemic ended, and the Inuit now make up a very small portion of tuberculous patients in Canada – 1.1 per cent in 1987–89. Their rate of infection, though still high, is lower than that of either the native Indians or Canadians born in Asia.[1] That the rates in the Inuit population have dropped so markedly compared with the appalling rates at the mid-century, when they were considered to have the highest incidence of TB in the world, is undoubtedly due to the massive effort put out by Health and Welfare in the thirty years or so following 1945. In the face of such a success, it may seem mere carping to criticize its programs, particularly when one considers the horrors that have been deliberately inflicted on ethnic minorities or on dissident groups by governments throughout the world and through all history. People do not even need to be ethnically different or conquered or dissident to be grossly ill-treated – as the conditions of child labourers in the nineteenth-century mines and mills, for instance, show. They just have to be vulnerable and to have something that more powerful people want, whether this is land, labour, sex, or anything else.

But these events took place in the mid-twentieth century in a democracy that prides itself on its help to the needy of the world and its championship of human rights in other less enlightened countries. All things considered, the government should have done better, not perhaps in bringing the epidemic under control, but in terms of minimizing the inevitable suffering of the Inuit community and some of the harmful social consequences of the medical programs. It is not quite a case of "the operation was successful but the patient died," for the Inuit community is very much alive and well. But as Glenn Tinder points out, according to Western political philosophy, "governments – indeed, all persons who wield power – must treat individuals with care. This can mean various things – for example, that individuals are to be fed and sheltered when they are destitute, listened to when they speak ... It always means that human beings are not to be treated like the things we use and discard or just leave lying about."[2] In short, governments are there to serve the people, not the other way around.

This, perhaps, is the nub of the criticism. While the treatment programs may have been essential and were perhaps the only way possible at the time to control the epidemic, the manner in which they were planned and implemented left much to be desired. In the record of the government's actions, several features stand out on the negative side of the ledger:

- the perpetual stalling and inaction of the department responsible for Inuit affairs during the 1930s and 1940s in the face of requests for help and continual warnings from the medical fraternity and others about the lamentable health situation in the Arctic;
- the arbitrariness and dictatorial nature of the Eastern Arctic Patrol evacuations in the late 1940s and 1950s, when the people were treated much like serfs or sick animals;
- the lack of any attempt to prepare the patients for their entry into the alien southern life, to provide for their dependents left up north, or to ensure future communication between the relatives and both patients and doctors;
- the poor record keeping and the confusion and apparent lack of planning at Health and Welfare (H&W) in the allocation of patients to particular hospitals;
- the arbitrary "disposal" of children from the hospitals, and the inadequate clothing and care taken when returning patients home;
- the lack of support systems for the patients in hospital, so that they were left with inadequate or, often, no interpretation services, no cash for incidentals, and no channels of outside (nonmedical) support, such as an ombudsman or patient's friend to help replace the psychological comfort that a family would normally provide;
- the internal government service rivalries between H&W on the one hand, and DRD and Northern Affairs on the other, and between H&W and the missions;
- the refusal of H&W to develop hospital treatment in the North, despite the presence of the mission hospitals and some mining company and American military hospitals already operating there.

Most of these criticisms apply to conditions during the earlier years of the hospitalization program, conditions that were modified as time went on. But they should not have happened in the first place and, having happened, they should have been far more speedily redressed.

Why did a responsible government service, made up of generally well-intentioned and presumably intelligent people, so mishandle things? The usual explanation put forward is that the formidable geography of the area, the lack of technical development and communication systems in the North at the time, and the extremely difficult working conditions made it impossible to behave in any other way. Of course conditions were very difficult in the Arctic, and particularly so for the visiting southerners on, for instance, the *C.D. Howe*. But the mere fact that the handling of the programs improved in the late 1950s and 1960s without any change in the Arctic weather and geography – and with minimal increase, if any, of the technical development available – underlines the hollowness of this excuse. Military and mining operations, including some medical facilities, had been successfully established in many places by the 1950s. When the will and the money were there, the difficulties could certainly be overcome. The real causes of the programs' faults must lie elsewhere.

Perhaps the main reason was one of which many of the government workers may not even have been aware, because they were so much a part of it, so immersed in it, that it seemed entirely normal; namely, the prevailing colonial, paternalistic attitudes of the period in which they had been reared.[3] Nowadays, such attitudes have become so unacceptable to many people that even mentioning that they used to exist is sometimes seen as evidence that one has a racist attitude. Revisionist history is not confined to communist societies, nor are prejudice and racism limited to whites. But in the early part of the century, there was generally the smug – and ignorant – assumption among white societies that they were superior to the local people who lived off the land that the whites coveted; and that, in the case of the Arctic, they would bring the benefits of civilization to the Inuit.

In some technical respects, this was true, of course; and the Inuit, being no more stupid than other people, knew it. They knew many things much better than the southerners, but they did not possess either the modern medical knowledge or the facilities to cure themselves of the diseases which the Europeans had inadvertently brought them, and they were appreciative of the help they received. But they did have their own culture and society. They knew very well the factors on which their survival depended, and they knew how they wished to conduct their lives – and deaths – in their own land. If they had been consulted, if they had been presented with the possible alternative ways of dealing with the epidemic and been given the chance to consider what each alternative would mean to their community, to decide what they would prefer to have done, and to explain what they would need in order to enable the sick to accept any treatment offered, there might have been some delay – even some additional deaths, perhaps – but much suffering and bitterness could have been avoided. To some extent, this seems to have happened in Newfoundland.

The TB eradication program had many of the same weaknesses of later attempts by the industrialized countries and Western experts to help the poor nations of the world overcome their economic and environmental problems. Many aid organizations have tended to impose or advise solutions based on the donor nation's values and circumstances, and this has often led to more serious problems because the local circumstances, values, and behaviour have neither been fully understood nor accepted as valid. By the 1980s, this problem was recognized, as was reported in the 1987 World Commission on Environment and Development Report to the United Nations.[4] The author of this report, Gro Brundtland, found that the most effective and least damaging way of providing help was through small, local, village cooperative-type programs, which depended on the input of those needing help and which had a wide-spectrum appreciation of the interrelationship of many aspects of life.

The TB eradication program for the Inuit was of a type almost exactly opposite to that later recommended by Brundtland. It was imposed by outside government experts, with no local community input; it required only passive acceptance on the part of those to be helped, and it took account only of the specific physical medical problem. To some extent the Welfare Division's efforts modified this pattern, but the values and circumstances of the Inuit, and the importance of other aspects of their lives to the solution of their problem with tuberculosis, were virtually disregarded by the medical authorities.

Although the Brundtland Report shows clearly that this pattern has been repeated in other circumstances by other professions, the medical profession may be particularly prone to adopt this style because of the excessive authority with which our society has generally invested it. We may argue with other experts from whom we seek advice – about our cars, our homes, our finances, for instance. But when we fall ill or are afraid for our lives or our health, our need has a much more personal urgency and we tend to accept whatever help we can get. We have, to some extent, abrogated our own responsibility for our health and medical treatment to the physicians, who, being human, assume power along with the responsibility – and, being human, once they have acquired power, they are loth to give it up.

This attitude is particularly marked when patients do not pay the doctors directly for their services. In our materialistic society, it is the converse of the old adage that "he who pays the piper calls the tune": he who does *not* pay the piper does *not* call the tune, even if he is the one who has to dance to it. This general societal attitude affects doctor-patient relationships even when the patient pays indirectly through publicly funded schemes such as medicare. It operates more strongly when it is clear that the patients are not contributing at all to the medical costs, for example, in the case of welfare patients or senior citizens in many plans. However flourishing and competent the Inuit were in living off the land in the Arctic, because of their cashless economy they were in the situation of indigent welfare patients as far as the doctors on the patrols and in the hospitals down south were concerned. Once they left their own environment, the Inuit lost their independent status and all possibility of controlling their fate or even of returning home without government help and, therefore, permission. Inevitably, they were totally in the power of the authorities around them.

As well, the Canadian medical establishment, which dominated all the decision-making bodies concerned with the provision of medical services in the North around 1945–55,[5] was, with a few exceptions, perhaps too focused on the purely physical aspects of disease, unwilling to admit the importance of environment and the emotions in the treatment and progress of disease. Even some army psychiatrists in World War II downplayed the effects of environment in favour of the adequacy or otherwise of a soldier's basic personality, and consequently they categorized the majority of neuropsychiatric battle casualties as the result of a neurotic condition predating enlistment rather than the result of experiences in battle.[6] Many of the H&W physicians had lately been in the armed forces and were accustomed to ordering their patients about and deciding on their treatment without their decisions being questioned.

Lastly, the old frustrations of the doctors in the days when the northern administration's policies – or lack of them – prevailed in the government's medical provisions for the Arctic may have played a part in H&W's apparent determination to thwart the department at every opportunity once it gained control after the war. The senior doctors in the Northern Health Service did not seem to be willing to listen to any advice from the nonmedical community or to acknowledge the possibility that they themselves might be wrong.

All of this was bad enough, but the problems were compounded by the sloppy record keeping and the apparent ignorance of the North of many of the workers to whom the actual operation of the programs was left. This was not necessarily the workers' fault. It was poor administration on the part of the upper levels of the Northern Health Service. With better systems in place and a greater awareness of the conditions and the Inuit's life up north, incidents such as people being sent home with inadequate clothing, or sent to the wrong settlement, or being unable to be located in any hospital, or being left as the single Inuit patient in a hospital, would surely not have happened. The doctors may have been poor administrators, arbitrary in their decisions, not paying enough attention to aspects other than the physical health of their patients; but their intentions were certainly good, and they probably did what they genuinely thought was right, given the circumstances in which they found themselves. Most nurses and doctors undoubtedly worked hard and with compassion for their Inuit patients.

Nor was H&W entirely to blame for the faults of the programs. The prewar northern administrators, with their inaction and heel dragging (and possibly even their suppression or conversion of unwelcome information)[7] set the scene for the H&W onslaught. In 1945 the department was still trying to justify its by then indefensible position, apparently more concerned with protecting its own reputation than with planning how to cooperate with the new power of H&W in the service of the people for whom it had been made responsible by the federal government.

Its officers were subject to the influences of their upbringing in the colonialist period, and many of them, too, had served in the armed forces in either World War I or World War II – for instance, Major McKeand, who was superintendent of the Arctic and chief government agent on the Eastern Arctic Patrol for many years. These men were not averse to authoritarian programs and did not hesitate to institute them when they thought it necessary, as in the dog-tag Eskimo identification numbers system. They and the RCMP had been running the North for so long, often doubling their roles in the department or the RCMP by holding the dominant positions in the Council of the Northwest Territories – disposing of "crown lands" for mining, military, or other southern concerns with little if any regard to the people who lived on them – that they doubtless expected to keep it that way. They had a natural resistance to the new mood of respect for *all* people's rights and needs that gathered momentum after World War II and included the H&W doctors' drive to provide an effective medical service to the native peoples.

Despite its disapproval of the aggressive health programs of H&W, Northern Affairs was driven into action on behalf of its clientele only by the outcries of others – notably, Bishop Marsh, the Oblate and Anglican missionaries, a few fieldworkers such as Leo Manning, and outside observers who were visiting or working temporarily in the North. Only when the department was forced into developing the miniscule welfare service and, perhaps inadvertently, engaged as its chief an activist who drew others of like mind into the service, did the impetus for change begin to come from within the department itself.

Nor can the politicians in the federal government escape blame. However much the staff in the public service may manipulate their ministers, devise and implement plans, and, in effect, rule the country, it is the politicians whom we, the people, elect to govern us as we would wish. And it is they who should initiate the policies, oversee the way in which the policies are implemented, and bear responsibility for the results. Theoretically, if the policies and programs are good (that is, if we, the people, approve of them), the politicians will be rewarded with re-election; and if the policies do not meet our approval, the politicians will be out of government next time around. We have no such control over the public servants; it is up to the politicians to direct them. If our elected representatives do not direct the public service in the way we want, we cease to be any sort of a democracy.

Looking back at the course of events, without having examined cabinet documents or any political records at all, it seems to me that our federal politicians of the time had even less concern for the native people of the Arctic than had the public servants. The Inuit cast no votes and carried nó weight on the national or international stage. When the politicians thought of the Far North, they were far more likely to consider the interests of the mining companies, the fur traders, and their international military agreements than the wishes of the local inhabitants, of whom they were probably only barely aware. It is typical that when RCMP officers were decorated after exploits such as the patrol from Hudson Bay to Coppermine during World War I, their Inuit guides and companions were ignored. Yet the police could not have operated without their help.

But even the politicians had to take notice eventually, and it is perhaps significant that improvements in the programs began to be effected after Bishop Marsh's direct approach to the prime minister, despite the sudden rush of senior H&W and Northern Affairs staff to present a united front to their ministers. Undoubtedly, the politicians must share the responsibility for any faults in the programs, especially since they allocated the money that was essential for the programs' existence. And while H&W needed the generous funds it was given, the imbalance between its funding and that accorded Northern Affairs and its predecessors may have helped contribute to the scarcity of support programs for the Inuit patients, since H&W was focused almost entirely on the purely medical treatment.

So much for the negative aspects of the TB eradication program. Were there any positive aspects, besides the major and all-important one of saving the people physically from the ravages of the epidemic? Indeed there were, even in the development and application of the programs.

First, however arbitrary the doctors were and however insensitive to the feelings of their clientele, they were determined to provide the best physical treatment available at the time for whatever ailed their patients. When H&W took over, the treatment of tuberculosis involved long stays in sanatoria and, often, radical surgery, and this the doctors provided for the Inuit with the same care they would give any other Canadians. When drug therapies became available, they switched to them, gradually developing suitable dosages and combinations, and introduced the system of supervised drug therapy in the settlements and the BCG immunization program. Although the doctors argued with the department and the churches about costs, they never seem to have limited treatments for patients because of the expense, which was heavy.

Secondly, individual hospitals bent over backwards to accommodate the special needs of the Inuit patients, though it may not have seemed so to the patients at the time. The staff were handicapped by the language difficulty and by their imperfect knowledge of their patients' culture and of conditions in the Arctic, and perhaps by their own rigid training and systems. But much learning went on in both groups, and the southerners' knowledge and appreciation of the Far North and its people expanded as a consequence.

Thirdly, as the social-activist welfare attitudes became stronger, the worst features of the x-ray surveys and the Eastern Arctic Patrol were modified until an acceptable system was in place, given the exigencies of the voyage. It was, in any event, quite an achievement to send a fully equipped and staffed hospital ship annually through such difficult waters and on such a schedule, particularly if the bulk of her crew was as inexperienced as was alleged.

On the human side, the record shows the greatness of heart of many of the people involved – of the workers, on the one hand, the doctors, nurses, RCMP, missionaries, traders, welfare officers, able seamen, flyers, and others; and, on the other hand, of the Inuit themselves. The accounts of life in the Arctic hamlets in the 1950s show how much endurance, determination, good humour, courage, and even self-sacrifice the workers needed to make their skills available to the Inuit, even if they had other reasons for being in the North and other obligations. Similarly, the material collected through interviews with the Inuit themselves and with southerners who worked on their behalf reveals the vastness of the Inuit's tolerance of the intruders, their general nonaggressive cooperation, and their acceptance of the chances and misfortunes of life, which much impressed some southerners, who were accustomed to a more competitive, unforgiving society. The Rev. Brian Burrows, for example, recalled with admiration an Inuk mother, who had just given birth to still-born twins, herself comforting the doctor who had delivered the babies. Many of the patients seem to have shown a greatness of spirit that somehow helped them survive illness, indignity, and years of exile without losing their essential tolerance, humanity, and independence.

As far as the side effects of the treatment went, the southern hospitalization program certainly introduced the Inuit to another way of life very speedily. It was a form of total immersion and it applied to a wide range of ordinary people, rather than being a gentle intermittent study session conducted in their own environment for a few gifted students or selected leaders of the community. Like total immersion language courses, it worked very well for some, could barely be tolerated by others, and for some was stressful in the extreme. It undoubtedly produced great culture shock, which was particularly hard for the older people to absorb successfully, but at least it was egalitarian, and it was probably a boon to many younger people. The southerners and their technological society were invading the Far North anyway, indeed, were already there. This may have been as good a way as any that a careless, inactive government could have devised to introduce the strangers and their values to the Inuit as a whole – to see us in something approaching our own setting and therefore to understand us better. The whites in the Far North were a self-selected group and did not really represent our southern society. Down south, the Inuit had more opportunity to see us as we are, warts and all.

The need for occupation and communication in the hospitals eventually stimulated the formation of the academic classes, particularly for the children, and the handicraft and carving at which the Inuit were already expert. At the same time, these spread into the settlements through the efforts of such people as the Houstons and, together with the cooperative movement which was largely started by the welfare workers from Northern Affairs, became a major economic and employment activity in the Arctic. Inuit art and sculpture have since flourished and become world famous, and some maintain this is the only characteristic Canadian art, though Indian artists and admirers of the Group of Seven may disagree.

The schooling begun in the hospitals had to be continued when the young patients returned home, and this stimulated Northern Affairs to develop local education. For many young patients, and for those in their teens or twenties, the stay down south opened up opportunities which they might never have otherwise had. Most returned to the North, but some young adults stayed in the South for a time to learn more or to work for the government, for instance as translators. The experiences of these people may have helped their community develop the political skills needed in the modern Canada into which the Inuit were inevitably being drawn.

Sometimes the southerners were more critical about our way of life and more concerned about its impact on the Inuit than the Inuit themselves were. Alma Houston was one such person, as she explained in an interview for *Business Quarterly*:

One man told me: "You white people feel very guilty about a lot of things that have happened up here." I said, "I guess we do because it was so beautiful when we first came." He replied: "Well, none of us would go back to it, you know. The business of going out hunting and knowing that if you didn't get that seal you were going to come back and face a really hungry family; that was something that was very bad for us."

Another told me back in 1955 after he had returned from a southern hospital that on the way to the airport he saw the factories and other signs of material progress and thought the white man must have been very good to have done this. I replied: "No, we are very materialistic, we do everything wrong. It's your culture that's beautiful." And I believed what I said. "No," he replied, "we're a people asleep."[8]

I do not believe that a people asleep could have devised ways of surviving, let alone developed a spiritual culture, in so harsh and unforgiving an environment as the Arctic. But many Inuit were undoubtedly very glad to be introduced to southern material goods and to have the chance to make their lives more secure and comfortable. Given their philosophy, perhaps they accepted the inevitability of a loss of some sort in exchange. All life is a balance, and there are two sides to every experience. It just depends what one makes of it. As a southerner, I cannot presume to suggest what the

Inuit have really made of the events of this traumatic period in their history. I can only look on from the outside. But there are some conclusions that, as a Canadian, I might suggest that we as a whole could draw from the events.

First, even the best-intentioned people can go wrong if given too much power; and in view of human greed and lust for power, the ordinary people must always be vigilant to defend their rights and freedom. Even in a democratic society, there must be mechanisms in place to assert and protect the rights of the individual versus the state. Secondly, specialists of any profession should not be given sole authority for decision making in public programs, even in their own specialty. Every major program has much wider effects than a single profession can envisage, and these need to be taken into account. Thirdly, central governments, particularly in a country as large and varied as Canada, should not impose programs or solutions on any group without that group's genuine participation in the decision making and implementation of the programs, except on a limited basis in situations of extreme emergency.

Lastly, in any program involving the subjugation of individual rights to the collective good – such as the isolation of infectious patients in the TB program – great care should be taken, in particular, to:

- inform the people about the authority and the reasons for the actions, and about the alternatives and their consequences;
- ensure that the reasonable needs and fears of the individuals are met; for instance, provision for dependents, communication links with families, explanation of what is to happen to the individuals and in what timeframe, and provision of all the necessities of which the individuals are otherwise deprived through being in the program;
- keep immaculate records, and keep individuals and their families informed of progress, plans, and so on;
- provide an independent appeal/second-opinion mechanism.

In a country such as Canada – so large, so varied in geography and climate, made up of so many races, each with its own values and historical background, and with many different religions – it is very difficult for us to be knowledgeable about the whole country and really to know our neighbours, let alone care about their problems, unless they come into competition with us. Perhaps we should look more to the old value system that our First Peoples developed over thousands of years to help them survive in the Arctic: cooperation rather than confrontation, respect for intelligence rather than mere physical prowess, integration with nature, acceptance of the inevitable balance of life – night and day, warmth and cold, rest and activity, female and male, misfortune and hard times as well as success and comfort. Maybe such values are a fundamental aspect of our country itself, part of the Canadian heritage, as self-defining as Inuit sculpture or Indian totem poles or ice hockey. At least they seem to fit our image of ourselves as peacekeepers and aid givers on the international scene. Perhaps they would even help us to survive in the harsh world of the twenty-first century.

Appendices

Arctic Administration and Principal Events, 1870–1970

Year	Department responsible	Operational unit(s)	Relevant events	Year
1870	Interior (D.Int.)		Medical services supplied by missions and traders at some points during this period	1870
1873	"	NWMP – southern and western territories		
			Yukon Territory proclaimed	1898
1904	"	NWMP became RNWMP and moved north		
1905	"	RNWMP	North-West Territory proclaimed	1905
1920	"	RNWMP became RCMP	RNWMP, missions, and HBC carrying out some admin	
1922	" (reorganized)	NWT&Y branch (O.S. Finnie); Eskimo Affairs Unit plus RCMP	Northern Health Service (NHS) begun (Dr Livingstone)	1922
			Eastern Arctic Patrol (EAP) begun	
1927	"	NWT&Y branch	Some doctors in mission hospitals funded by D.Int.	1927
			Indian Health Service (IHS) started by Dept of Indian Affairs (Dr Stone)	
1931	"	Dominion Lands Board (H.E. Hume); NWT section		
1934	"	Lands, NWT&Y branch (J.L. Turner); NWT section		

Year	Department responsible	Operational unit(s)	Relevant events	Year
1936	Mines and Resources (DMR) (formed from D.Int.; Indian Affairs; Mines; Immigration and Colonization)	Lands, Parks, and Forests branch (R.A. Gibson); Bureau of NWT&Y Affairs; Eastern Arctic Div. (D.L. McKeand, sup.)	Indian Health Services (including Eskimos) replaces NHS and IHS (Dr Stone)	1936
			Dr Moore director of IHS	1939
1943	"	"	Dr Wherrett's survey	1943
			Dept of National Health and Welfare (H&W) formed (Dr Brock Chisholm)	1945
			IHS transferred to H&W	
			Advisory committee for the control and prevention of TB in Indians	
1946	"	" (J.G. Wright, sup. of Eastern Arctic Div.)	X-ray surveys and southern hospitalization program begun	1946
1947	"	Lands and Development Services (R.A. Gibson); Arctic Division (J.G. Wright)	Newfoundland joins Confederation. Labrador Inuit still serviced by IGA and Newfoundland, but IHS contributes cash for hospitalized patients	1949
1950	Resources and Development (DRD)	Development Services branch (R.A. Gibson); Northern Admin Service; Arctic Division	Indian Affairs branch transferred to Dept of Citizenship and Immigration	1950
1951	"	Northern Admin and Lands branch (G.E.B. Sinclair); Arctic Serv.; Education and Welfare Services		
1953	Northern Affairs and National Resources (NANR)	NA&L branch (F.J.G. Cunningham); Arctic Division	Advisory Committee on Northern Development begun (to coordinate work of all departments in the North)	1953
1954	"	" (B.G. Sivertz takes over Arctic Div.)	Mounting criticism of EAP and services for the Inuit	1954

Year	Department responsible	Operational unit(s)	Relevant events	Year
			IHS becomes Indian and Northern Health Service (INHS)	1955
			Centralization of hospitalized Inuit patients begun	
			Rudnicki appointed; Welfare Section begun	
1956–57	"	NA&L branch (B.G. Sivertz, 1957); Arctic Div. (R.A.J. Phillips); Welfare Section (W. Rudnicki)	Robertson both DM/NANR and commissioner of the NWT	1956–57
			Cunningham deputy commissioner of NWT and ADM/NANR	
1959	"	Northern Admin branch (B.G. Sivertz); Educational, Industrial, and Welfare divs. (W. Rudnicki)	Field administrative operations offices set up for Mackenzie and Arctic regions	1959
			NA admin taken off EAP; welfare officer becomes senior NA officer; senior MO becomes O.i/c EAP	1960
1962	NANR given two new ADMS; Northern Admin branch under ADM for Northern Affairs	"	NHS put under Medical Services branch at H&W (director general, Dr Moore)	1962
1963	"	" (R.A.J. Phillips to NA branch)	Gradual transfer of responsibility for services for Ungava Inuit to Quebec	1963
1964	"	" (F.A.G. Carter to NA branch)	Both NA branch and Advisory Committee report to ADM/NA	1964
			Dr Moore retires 1965	
1966	Indian Affairs and Northern Development (DIAND) – three programs: Indian Affairs; National and Historical Parks; Northern Development	Northern Development; NA branch (C.M. Bolger) and Advisory Committee	Indian Affairs branch moved to DIAND from Dept of Citizenship and Immigration	1966
			Yellowknife made capital of NWT; transfer of local government functions and public service from federal to territorial level begun	1967

Year	Department responsible	Operational unit(s)	Relevant events	Year
1968–69	DIAND reorganized as functions transferred to NWT government	Northern Devel. Program (ADM/J.H. Gordon, 1968; J.B. Bergevin, 1969)		
1970	DIAND responsible for functions remaining with federal government	" (ADM/A.D. Hunt, 1970) Indian/Eskimo Affairs program	Transfer of most functions and public servants to NWT government completed; federal programs in Arctic Quebec to Indian/Eskimo Affairs program; NWT government takes over Eastern Arctic and islands	1970

Interviews

WITH ALEXANDRA GRYGIER

Mini Aodla Freeman	Edmonton, Alta, November 1988
Dr O. Schaefer	Edmonton, Alta, November 1988
Elva Taylor	Edmonton, Alta, November 1988
Dr Demetrius Todosijczuk, CSPulmD, PQ	Edmonton, Alta, November 1988
Marie Uviluq (not taped)	Yellowknife, NWT, November 1988
Prof. R.G. (Bob) Williamson, CM	Saskatoon, Sask., November 1988

WITH THE AUTHOR

The Hon. Titus Allooloo, MLA	Ottawa, Ont., October 1990
Appeeya	Pangnirtung, NWT, September 1988
Dr B. Brett	Ottawa, Ont., March 1988
The Rev. B. Burrows	Hamilton, Ont., October 1989
Dr K. Butler	Ottawa, Ont., March 1988
Fr Charles Choque, OMI (not taped)	Ottawa, Ont., March 1990
Charlie Crow, former MLA	St Marys, Ont., December 1989
Elizabeth	Iqaluit, NWT, October 1988
Dr H.T. Ewart (not taped)	Dundas, Ont., May 1987
Leo Flaherty (not taped)	Toronto, Ont., November 1989
Jacob Jaypoody	Clyde River, NWT, September 1988
Joanna Kautaq	Clyde River, NWT, September 1988
Lena	Pangnirtung, NWT, October 1988
Betty M. Marwood, MSW	Manotick, Ont., March and May 1988
F.J. (Bud) Neville	Ottawa, Ont., January 1987
Abraham Okpik	Iqaluit, NWT, September 1988
Ralph Ritcey	Ottawa, Ont., January 1987
Graham Rowley, CM (not taped)	Ottawa, Ont., January 1987
Walter Rudnicki	Ottawa, Ont., March and May 1988
Joanasie Salomonie	Cape Dorset, NWT, September 1988

Alex. Spalding   Toronto, Ont., July 1989
Thomas Suluk, former MP   Ottawa, Ont., March 1988
A.L. Young (not taped)   Kitchener, Ont., March 1987

The following informants were contacted by the author by telephone. The conversations were not taped.
Dr Noah Carpenter   Comox, BC, September 1990
Molly Gibbard   Hamilton, Ont., October 1989
Ivan Mowatt   Salt Spring Island, BC, September 1990
R.A.J. Phillips, CM   Cantley, Que., March 1988
Freda Richards   Hamilton, Ont., June 1987
B.G. Sivertz, OBE   Victoria, BC, September 1990

Hospitals to which Inuit Were Sent, 1940s to 1960s

NORTHWEST TERRITORIES
All Saints, Aklavik
Immaculate Conception, Aklavik
Ste-Thérèse, Chesterfield Inlet
General Hospital, Fort Smith
St Luke's, Pangnirtung
U.S. Army Hospital, Southampton Island
Red Cross Hospital, Yellowknife

NOVA SCOTIA
Dartmouth Mental Hospital, Dartmouth
Nova Scotia Hospital, Dartmouth
Children's Hospital, Halifax
Halifax Infirmary Hospital, Halifax
HMCS Stadacona, RCN Hospital, Halifax
Victoria General Hospital, Halifax
Miller Sanatorium, Kentville

NEWFOUNDLAND
Grenfell Mission Hospital, Cartwright
RCAF Hospital, Goose Bay
Grenfell Mission Hospital, Northwest River
Grenfell Mission Hospital, St Anthony
St Mary's Hospital, St Mary's
St John's San., St John's

QUEBEC
L'Hôpital du Sacré Coeur, Cartierville
Kateri Memorial, Caughnawaga

Sacred Heart, Caughnawaga
Ste-Justine, Caughnawaga
Alexandra, Montreal
Children's Memorial, Montreal
Grace Dart, Montreal
Julius Richardson Convalescent Home, Montreal
L'Hôtel Dieu, Montreal
Montreal General Hospital, Montreal
Notre-Dame, Montreal
Royal Victoria Hospital, Montreal
St Luke's, Montreal
Verdun Protestant, Montreal
Parc Savard (Quebec immigration hospital), Quebec City
Quebec Veterans', Quebec City
Quebec West, Quebec City
Roberval Hospital, Roberval
St Michael's, Roberval
Ste-Agathe San., Ste-Agathe
Laval, Ste-Foy
Veteran's Hospital, Ste-Foy

ONTARIO
Cochrane Hospital, Cochrane
Fort William San., Fort William
Muskoka Hospital, Gravenhurst
Mountain San. (now Chedoke Hospital), Hamilton
Moose Factory Indian Hospital, Moose Factory
Ste-Thérèse, Moosonee
Rideau Health Centre, Ottawa
Queen Alexandra San., London
Queen Mary Hospital for TB children, Toronto
Sunnybrook, Toronto
Toronto General, Toronto
Weston TB San., Toronto
Essex County San., Windsor

MANITOBA
Assiniboine, Brandon
Brandon Mental Hospital, Brandon
Brandon TB San., Brandon
Churchill Military Hospital, Churchill
Fisher River Indian Hospital, Fisher River
Ninette TB San., Ninette

Norway House Indian Hospital, Norway House
St Boniface, St Vital
Dynevor Indian Hospital, Selkirk
Selkirk Mental Hospital, Selkirk
Selkirk TB San., Selkirk
Clearwater Lake San., The Pas
St Anthony's, The Pas
Central TB Clinic, Winnipeg
D.A. Stewart Centre, Winnipeg
General Hospital, Winnipeg
King Edward, Winnipeg
King George, Winnipeg
Princess Elizabeth, Winnipeg
St Aman Centre, Winnipeg
Winnipeg Municipal Hospital, Winnipeg

ALBERTA
Central Alberta San., Calgary
Alberta Mental Hospital, Edmonton
Charles Camsell, Edmonton
Eberhart Memorial, Edmonton
Edmonton General Hospital, Edmonton
Misericordia, Edmonton
Oliver Hospital (now Alberta Hospital), Edmonton
Saint Joseph's, Edmonton
University of Alberta Hospital, Edmonton

Sources: National Archives of Canada, RG85, vols. 1128, 1129, 1474, 1475, and 1872; and Government of the Northwest Territories, Department of Health, Medical Patient Search Project, *Summary: Final Report*, 1991.

NANR *"Standard Eskimo Discharge Kit"*

GENERAL ISSUE

1	Parka	1 each
	(The following material may be obtained from the Northern Administration Branch for manufacture of this article in hospital)	
	– 3 yds duffle for one man's parka and 3½ yds coloured drill for one man's parka	
	– 3½ yds duffle for one woman's parka and 5 yds coloured drill for one woman's parka	
2	Rubber boots – sheep-skin lined or native made boots (mukluks might be made in hospital out of tanned hides)	1 pair each
3	Duffle socks (duffle socks are to be made if possible in hospital from scraps of material left over from parkas)	1 pair each
4	Woollen socks – heavy gray	2 pairs each
5	Leather mitts – as in Eaton's Catalogue – Fall & Winter, 1956–57, p. 8, 1-M-8055	1 pair each
6	Liners for mitts (woollen mitts)	1 pair each
7	Kit Bag	1 each
8	Sleeping Bag (patient's disc number to be marked on sleeping bag in indelible ink in hospital)	1 each

MALE ISSUE

1	Underwear shirts, woollen (long sleeves)	2 each
2	Underwear drawers, woollen	2 pairs each
3	Shirts, flannelette	2 each
4	Cardigan, woollen	1 each

5 Trousers, heavy tweed	1 pair each
6 Over pants or jeans (to wear over trousers)	1 pair each
7 Helmet – leather	1 each
8 Belt or braces	1 each
9 Boots – leather, Army type with rubber heels	1 pair each
10 Underwear, light – shorts and shirt	2 sets

FEMALE ISSUE

1 Underwear shirts, woollen	2 each
2 Underwear drawers, woollen	2 pairs each
3 Slacks, ankle length	1 pair each
4 Bloomers, all wool	2 pairs each
5 Brassieres, all cotton	2 each
6 Stockings, lisle	2 pairs each
7 Garter belt	
8 Dresses, cotton one piece	2 each
9 Sweater coat	1 each
10 Scarf, head	1 each
11 Shoes	1 pair each
12 Underwear, light	2 sets each

BOYS' ISSUE

1 Underwear shirts, woollen	2 each
2 Underwear drawers, woollen	2 pairs each
3 Shirts, flannelette	2 each
4 Trousers, heavy and jeans	1 pair each
5 Sweater coat	1 each
6 Belt or braces	1 each
7 Helmet – leather	1 each
8 Shoes	1 pair
9 Underwear, light	2 sets

GIRLS' ISSUE

1 Woollen vests	2 each
2 Woollen drawers	2 pairs each
3 Bloomers	2 pairs each
4 Hose, black or fawn	2 pairs each
5 Dresses	2 each
6 Sweater coat	1 each
7 Toque or beret	1 each
8 Shoes	1 pair each
9 Underwear, light	2 sets each

BABY'S ISSUE
Very young babies should be supplied with a complete layette, including suitable bunting, extra blankets and any other items necessary to protect the child against extremes of cold.

March 19, 1957

Source: Walter Rudnicki, personal files.

Notes

INTRODUCTION

1 See National Archives of Canada (NA), RG85, 362: 201-1(30), a survey of "Settlements in the Northwest Territories" prepared by G.W. Rowley for the Advisory Committee on Northern Development, 1954. Among settlements in Inuit country this survey listed only Aklavik as having a larger permanent population (400); but Aklavik, with two mission hospitals, was also home to whites and Loucheux Indians. Four other settlements had sizable trading populations, or groups living on the land nearby and coming in to trade: Cape Dorset (399), Baker Lake (393), Pangnirtung (568), and Inukjuak (392). But the permanent Inuit population of each of these settlements was 100 or less. See also the *Hamilton Spectator*, 19 April 1989.
2 *North* 9, no. 2 (March–April 1962): 45.

CHAPTER ONE

1 "Canadian Discoveries & Inventions," *Horizon Canada* 9, no. 104 (1987): 2496.
2 Some authorities estimate the rate as high as two in 1,000. See A.S. Brancker et al., "A Statistical Chronicle of Tuberculosis in Canada: Part I. From the Era of Sanatorium Treatment to the Present," *Health Reports 1992* 4, no. 2, Statistics Canada, cat. 82-003, 107.
3 Pat Bayer, "Canada's 50 Year Old Battle against the 'White Plague,'" *Saturday Night*, 17 November 1945, 34.
4 Brancker et al., "Statistical Chronicle of Tuberculosis in Canada: Part I," 114.
5 D.A. Enarson, "Risk of Tuberculosis in Canada: Implications for Priorities in Programs Directed at Specific Groups," *Canadian Journal of Public*

Health 28 (September–October 1987): 305–8. See also A.S. Brancker et al., "A Statistical Chronicle of Tuberculosis in Canada: Part II. Risk Today and Control," *Health Reports 1992* 4, no. 3, Statistics Canada, cat. 82-003, 285.

6 G.J. Wherrett, *Tuberculosis in Canada* (Ottawa: Royal Commission on Health Services, 1965), chap. 2.

7 *Everyman's Encyclopaedia* (London: J.M. Dent & Sons, 1968), 12:137–9.

8 Dr J.F. McLellan, district veterinarian, Agriculture Canada, personal communications, June 1990 and January 1992.

9 For a fuller description from the patient's point of view, see L.K. Ryan, "Mystic Order of the Bug," *Maclean's Magazine*, 15 November 1941, 30–3; L. Walters, "I Conquered TB," *Maclean's Magazine*, 1 March 1943, 26–7; and J.P.D. McGinnis, "The White Plague in Calgary: Sanatorium Care in Southern Alberta," *Alberta History* 28, no. 4 (Autumn 1980): 1–15.

10 Brancker et al., "Statistical Chronicle of Tuberculosis in Canada: Part I," 110.

11 F.E. Mason, "Protection from TB Is Given by New Vaccine," *Saturday Night*, 30 August 1947, 9.

12 "The Development of B.C.G. (Bacillus Calmette Guérin) and Its Use in Indian Health Services," *IHS: Director's Newsletter*, December 1954, 15–17.

13 G.J. Wherrett, *The Miracle of the Empty Beds* (Toronto: University of Toronto Press, 1977), 87.

14 S.J. Hawkins, "Streptomycin in Tuberculosis," *Health*, November–December 1950, 19, 34.

15 See, for instance, A. Grant, "Give Them Jobs They Can Do," *Health*, May–June 1950, 10–11; and R.R. Trail, "An Industrial Colony for the Treatment of Tuberculosis," *Health*, September–October 1950, 14.

16 L. Postill, "Bed's Eye View," *Maclean's Magazine*, 1 November 1946, 40–1. See also "Some Psychological Aspects of Tuberculosis," *IHS: Director's Newsletter*, December 1952, 3–10.

17 B. McKone, "Post-sanatorium Rehabilitation," *Canadian Nurse* 44 (December 1948): 971–3.

18 B. Hellyar, "Approach to the Patient," *Canadian Nurse* 44 (December 1948): 974–6.

19 *American Health*, quoted in *Globe and Mail*, 25 March 1992; and "TB Emergency Declared," *Globe and Mail*, 24 April 1993.

20 Brancker et al., "Statistical Chronicle of Tuberculosis in Canada: Part I," 122, and "Part II," 277–92.

CHAPTER TWO

1 The Inuit use the word Inuuk for two people, but in this text, for simplicity's sake, the word Inuit is used whenever more than one person is referred to. For one person, the word Inuk is used.

2 "Northern News," *Arctic*, June 1954, 52–5.
3 *Native Languages of the* NWT, Northwest Territories Information, September 1984.
4 Environment Canada, personal communication, April 1990.
5 G.W. Rowley, *What Are Eskimos?* (Ottawa: Information Canada, 1971), 3.
6 Ibid., 5.
7 Darrell de Bow gives the measurements as 15–20 feet in diameter and 8–10 feet high. See "There's No Downpayment on an Igloo," *Maclean's Magazine*, 15 December 1950, 18–19, 52–3.
8 Abraham Okpik, "What Do the Eskimo People Want?" *North* 7, no. 2 (March–April 1960): 38–42.
9 P. Freuchen, "Out of the Stone Age," *Beaver*, September 1951, 3–9.
10 Robert Williamson, interviews by Alexandra Grygier, Saskatoon, November 1988.
11 See, for instance, J.P. Moody with W. de Groot van Embden, *Arctic Doctor* (New York: Dodd, Mead, 1955); G.W. Rowley, "Settlement and Transportation in the Canadian North," *Arctic* 7, nos. 3/4 (1955): 336–42; IHS: *Director's Newsletter* from 1948 on (for example, J.P. Moody's "Patrol Report Feb.–Mar. 48" in *Newsletter*, July 1948); and *Northern Affairs Bulletin*, vols. 1–5 (1954–58).
12 Alex. Spalding, *Aivilik Adventure*, in press, and personal communication.
13 Otto Schaefer, "Medical Observations and Problems in the Canadian Arctic," *Canadian Medical Association Journal* 81 (15 August 1959): 248–9.
14 Ibid., 249.
15 Ibid.
16 Ibid.
17 Otto Schaefer, interview by Alexandra Grygier, Edmonton, November 1988.
18 R. Horley, "Story of my Trip to Nunoodjuak," IHS: *Director's Newsletter*, December 1954.
19 Betty Lee, *Lutiapik* (Toronto: Simon and Pierre, 1975), 128–35, 157–74.
20 Ibid., 134–5.
21 Ibid., 166.
22 Schaefer, "Medical Observations and Problems in the Canadian Arctic," 250.

CHAPTER THREE

1 *Everyman's Encyclopaedia* (London: J.M. Dent & Sons, 1968), 6:517.
2 See Peter C. Newman, *Company of Adventurers* (Markham: Penguin Books Canada, 1985).
3 P.A.C. Nichols, "Enter the European: The Fur Traders," *Beaver*, Winter 1954, 37–8.

4 "Relief in the East Arctic", IHS: *Director's Newsletter*, September 1947, 18–20.
5 Gavin White, "Canadian Apartheid," *Canadian Forum*, August 1951, 102–3.
6 Peter Freuchen, "Out of the Stone Age," *Beaver*, September 1951, 5.
7 See *Northern Affairs Bulletin*, 2, no. 4 (1955): 1; ibid., 2, no. 11 (1955): 7; ibid., 4, no. 1 (1957): 3–5; and ibid., 5, no. 2 (1958): 6.
8 For the details about the work of the Oblates in the Arctic, see Charles Choque, OMI, *75th Anniversary of the First Catholic Mission to the Hudson Bay Inuit* (Diocese of Churchill Hudson Bay, 1987), and *The Grey Nuns of Chesterfield Inlet, N.W.T.* (Diocese of Churchill Hudson Bay, 1989). See also *Aux Glaces Polaires* (Bulletin missionaire for Oblates of the Mackenzie), 1965–71; and *Eskimo* (quarterly bulletin for Oblates of Churchill Hudson Bay), 1955–67 and 1971–77.
9 Arthur Thibert, OMI, "Enter the European: The Roman Catholic Missionaries," *Beaver*, Winter 1954, 34–6.
10 For details of the work of the Anglican church in the Arctic, see D.B. Marsh, "Enter the European: The Anglican Missionaries," *Beaver*, Winter 1954, 31–3.
11 Missions Verkehrs Arbeitsgemeinschaft.
12 Matthew Fisher, "Veteran Arctic Priest Caught between Two Cultures," *Globe and Mail*, 12 December 1988.
13 *Northern Affairs Bulletin*, 4, no. 1 (1957): 2.
14 National Archives of Canada (NA), RG85, 1871: 550-1-2, Bishop Fleming to R.A. Gibson, deputy commissioner, NWT, 18 March 1944.
15 "Education in Canada's Northland," *Northern Affairs Bulletin* (suppt.), 2, no. 1 (1955): 1–10.
16 George Hunter, "Cathedral of the North," *Beaver*, December 1953, 38–42.
17 The other members of the party were the secretary of the Northwest Territories Council and replacements for the Royal Canadian Mounted Police.
18 Jenness noted: "The Eskimos themselves contributed, directly or indirectly, as much perhaps as 40 per cent of this expenditure through the taxes that the government levied on their furs."
19 Diamond Jenness, *Eskimo Administration*, vol. 2, *Canada*, technical paper 14 (Montreal: Arctic Institute of North America, 1964), 70.
20 Ibid., 71.

CHAPTER FOUR

1 K.J. Crowe, *A History of the Original Peoples of Northern Canada*, rev. ed. (Montreal: Arctic Institute of North America, McGill-Queen's University Press, 1991), 171.

2 Terry Cook, *Records of the Northern Affairs Program (RG 85)* (Ottawa: Public Archives of Canada, Federal Division, 1982), 1.
3 Ibid., 3.
4 Ibid., 8.
5 Diamond Jenness, *Eskimo Administration*, vol. 2, *Canada*, technical paper 14 (Montreal: Arctic Institute of North America, 1964), 71.
6 Henry A. Larsen, "My Beat in the Arctic," *Saturday Night*, 8 November 1952, 11, 22.
7 J.P. Moody, with W. de Groot van Embden, *Arctic Doctor* (New York: Dodd, Mead, 1955), 182–6.
8 Ibid., 192–3.
9 G. Graham-Cumming, "Northern Health Services," *Canadian Medical Association Journal* 100 (15 March 1969): 527–8.
10 National Archives of Canada (NA), RG85, 1871: 550–1(1A), "Policy Respecting the Operation of Hospitals in the N.W.T.," a precis made for the NWT council by the Department of Mines and Resources, 22 June 1943.
11 Individual public servants often occupied senior positions in both the department responsible for administering the North and the NWT council. For instance, during the late 1930s, R.A. Gibson was director of the Bureau of Northwest Territories and Yukon Affairs at DMR and was also deputy commissioner of the NWT. He was approached on Inuit matters by officials from other departments or organizations sometimes as wearing one hat, sometimes the other. Since the council of the NWT sometimes referred matters brought for its consideration to the department responsible for administering the north (that is, to some of its own members), one can see the possibilities of manipulation, concentration of power, and administrative confusion.
12 Mini Aodla Freeman, interview by Alexandra Grygier, Edmonton, November 1988.

CHAPTER FIVE

1 S. Grzybowski, K. Styblo, and E. Dorken, "Tuberculosis in Eskimos," *Tubercle* 57, no. 4, supp. (1976): S2.
2 Ibid.
3 Ibid.
4 The account of Dr Martin's experiences at Coppermine is based on material in the National Archives of Canada (NA), RG85, 1118: 100/145-1, as follows: extract of minutes of NWT council, 4 February 1931; cable, O.S. Finnie, D.Int., to R.D. Martin, Coppermine, 14 February 1931; memo with attachments, Martin to Finnie, 25 March 1931; Martin, "Resumé of Work at Coppermine," 29 March 1931.
5 NA, RG85, 1118: 1000/145-1, memo, Martin to Finnie.

6 NA, RG85, 1872: 552-1(1), memo, A.L. Cumming to R.A. Gibson, 17 May 1937.

7 Ibid.

8 Ibid.

9 Grzybowski, Styblo, and Dorken, "Tuberculosis in Eskimos," s2.

10 NA, RG85, 1872: 552-1(1), memo, Cumming to Gibson, 17 May 1937.

11 Ibid.

12 P.G. Nixon, "Early Administrative Developments in Fighting Tuberculosis among Canadian Inuit: Bringing State Institutions Back In," *Northern Review*, Winter 1988, 71.

13 NA, RG85, 1872: 552-1(1), memo, T.J. Orford to Gibson, 15 August 1939.

14 Ibid.

15 Ibid., see memo, D.L. McKeand to Gibson, 5 December 1939.

16 Ibid.

17 Ibid., Gibson to E. Bickerstaffe, Britannica Research Bureau, 17 February 1940. See also notations on p. 2 of McKeand's memo to Gibson, 5 December 1939; and memo, R. Millar to McKeand, 13 February 1940.

18 Nixon, "Early Administrative Developments," 73.

19 NA, RG85, 1871: 550-1(1A).

20 NA, RG85, 1872: 552-1(1), "Extract from Dr L.D. Livingstone's Report, dated at Aklavik, 1st October, 1943."

21 NA, RG85, 1871: 550-1 (1A), memo, McKeand to Gibson, 25 October 1943; notes on the back of memo, Gibson to McKeand, 26 October 1943; McKeand to Gibson, 28 October 1943; and memo, Gibson to McKeand, 1 November 1943.

22 Ibid., memo, McKeand to Gibson, 25 October 1943.

23 NA, RG85, 1872: 552-1(1), Millar to Gibson, 22 February 1944.

24 NA, RG85, 1871: 550-1(2), memo, McKeand to Gibson, 22 March 1944.

25 NA, RG85, 1872: 552-1(1), report, Falconer to Gibson (undated).

26 NA, RG85, 76: 201-1(19), memo, McKeand to Gibson, 6 January 1944.

27 Cited in P.E. Moore, "No Longer Captain: A History of Tuberculosis and Its Control Amongst Canadian Indians," *Canadian Medical Association Journal* 84 (May 1961): 1015.

28 Nixon, "Early Administrative Developments," 75.

29 Ibid., 75.

30 Ibid., 75–6.

31 Ibid., 76.

32 G.J. Wherrett, "Arctic Survey I. Survey of Health Conditions and Medical and Hospital Services in the North West Territories," *Canadian Journal of Economics and Political Science* 11, no. 1 (1945).

33 Ibid., 60.

34 NA, RG85, 1871: 550-1(2), J.G. Wright, 17 January 1945.

35 Ibid., "Synopsis of Arrangements made by the Northwest Territories Administration for the Medical Care of Eskimos" (undated).

CHAPTER SIX

1 See J.W. Anderson, "Peacetime Voyage," *Beaver*, December 1946: 44–7.

2 National Archives of Canada (NA), RG 85, 78: 201-1(22); see "Precis for NWT Council" (undated), file 5031-17959; and memo, A. Stevenson to R.A. Gibson, 4 October 1947.

3 Diamond Jenness, *Eskimo Administration*, vol. 2, *Canada*, technical paper 14 (Montreal: Arctic Institute of North America, 1964), 85.

4 See NA, RG85, 79: 201-1(24), schedule for inspection trip by plane; and NA, RG85, 78: 201-1(23), Gibson to Capt. G.A. Worth, RCN, 21 July 1948.

5 NA, RG85, 79: 201-1(25A), memo, J.G. Wright to M.A. Watson, DoT, 22 December 1950. See also A. Stevenson, "The Eastern Arctic Patrol," *Arctic* 4, no. 1 (1951): 70–1.

6 See *Northern Affairs Bulletin* 2, no. 10 (1955): 3; ibid., 3, no. 4 (1956): 7; ibid., 4, no. 7 (1957): 11; and NA, RG85, 362: 201–1 (30), report by Dr R.N. Simpson, 18 October 1954.

7 NA, RG85, 1872: 552-1(1), Noel Rawson to Gibson, 2 February 1946. See also NA, RG85, 1871: 550-1(2), "Synopsis of Arrangements Made by the Northwest Territories Administration for the Medical Care of Eskimos," (undated, but from content and file placement written in fall, 1945).

8 Personal communication, Dr R.A. Macbeth, 1990.

9 NA, RG85, 1872: 550-1(3), report by Dr Callaghan, 1 May 1949.

10 *IHS: Director's Newsletter*, December 1949.

11 NA, RG85, 178: 552-1-1(2), and *Arctic Circular* 4, no. 3 (1951): 45–7.

12 *IHS: Director's Newsletter*, November 1952, 2–9.

13 *The Camsell Mosaic* (Edmonton: Charles Camsell History Committee, 1985), 136.

14 Kathleen Dier, "Early Days," *Canadian Nurse* 80, no. 1 (January 1984): 22.

15 Ibid.

16 See Jenness, *Eskimo Administration* 2:144, and R.G. Robertson, "The Future of the North," *North* 8, no. 2 (March–April 1961): 13.

17 *Camsell Mosaic*, 1–10.

18 *IHS: Director's Newsletter*, September 1947, 1–4.

19 *IHS: Director's Newsletter*, November 1952, 16–21.

20 NA, RG85, 1872: 550-1(2A), Falconer to Gibson, April 1948.

21 See, for instance, NA, RG85, 1873: 552-1(2), Moore to G.E.B. Sinclair, DRD, 12 October 1951.

22 NA, RG85, 1872: 550-1(3), file M-34/12.48, Moore's circular.

23 NA, RG85, 1873: 564-2(1), correspondence between the vicariate apostolic of Hudson Bay and the NWT administration, March 1946; and between Moore and the deputy commissioner, NWT, March 1947. See also NA, RG85, 1873: 564-5(1), correspondence between the Diocese of the Arctic and the NWT administration.

24 Otto Schaefer, interview by A. Grygier, Edmonton, November 1988.

25 NA, RG85, 1474: 252-3(6), L.H. Nicholson, commissioner, RCMP, to R.G. Robertson, deputy minister, NANR, 30 November 1954.

26 NA, RG85, 1129: 252-3(1B). Gibson to Moore, 28 December 1949, and Moore's reply, 17 January 1950.

27 NA, RG85, 1129: 252-3(2), "Eskimos in Hospital."

28 See correspondence in NA, RG85, 1129: 252-3(2) and (2A). Some sanatoria, however, such as the Charles Camsell, were quoted as regularly sending reports back to the settlements. The Quebec Immigration Hospital at Parc Savard also regularly sent reports to DMR which were passed on to the settlements – at least, by December 1953; see NA, RG85, 1474: 252-3(5).

29 NA, RG85, 1129: 252-3(3). See also NA, RG85, 1474: 252-3(5), which contains IHS "Applications for Medical Treatment," "Tuberculosis Case History Summary," and "Advice of Discharge" forms for individual Inuit in hospital in 1953.

30 NA, RG85, 1475: 252-4(1), memo, J. Cantley to J.V. Jacobsen, 3 June 1953.

31 Ibid., "Eskimo Discharges from Hospitals," 12 August 1955.

32 NA, RG85, 362: 201-1(30). "Report of B.G. Sivertz," 27 August 1954; and Stanley Burke, "Canada's Arctic Ship Dirty and Inefficient," *Vancouver Sun*, 10 September 1954.

33 NA, RG85, 1474: 252-3(6), for Bishop Marsh's letter of 10 November 1954 enclosing "Cry the Beloved Eskimo" and the subsequent correspondence. All the quotations referred to on pp. 76–80 are from this file (covering the period November 1954 to August 1955), except those from "Cry the Beloved Eskimo," which have been slightly amended to accord with the text given in Donald B. Marsh and Winifred Marsh, *Echoes into Tomorrow* (1991).

34 See list of hospitals in the *Medical Patient Search Project: Summary–Final Report* (Government of the Northwest Territories, Department of Health, April 1991). See also NA, RG85, vol. 1128: file 252-3(1); vol. 1129, files 252-3(1B), 252-3(2), 252-3(2A), 252-3(3); vol. 1474, files 252-3(5), 252-3(6); vol. 1475: 252-4(1); and vol. 1872: 552-1(1), in all of which various hospitals are named as treating Inuit patients. Although, as early as 1947, a report refers to four "Eskimo girls" in training at Pangnirtung hospital (NA, RG85, 78: 201-1(22)), the "substantial numbers of Eskimos" promised for the staff by Dr Moore did not seem to materialize. The INHS *Director's Report* for 1957 shows six Inuit occupying INHS positions at 31 December 1956, out of a total nonprofessional staff of 1,244.

35 S. Grzybowski, K. Styblo, and E. Dorken, "Tuberculosis in Eskimos," *Tubercle* 57, no. 4, supp. (1976): S10.

36 NA, RG85, 1873: 552-1(2), Moore to H.A. Young.

37 Grzybowski, Styblo, and Dorken, "Tuberculosis in Eskimos," S10.

38 See H. Brian Brett, "A Synopsis of Northern Medical History," *Canadian Medical Association Journal* 100 (15 March 1969): 521–5; and Jenness, *Eskimo Administration* 2:86–7.

39 NA, RG85 (Int. 98), 178: 552-1-1(2). See also IHS *Annual Report* for 1955 and 1956, and INHS *Director's Report* from 1957–58 to 1960–61.

40 See Robertson, "Future of the North"; and G.J. Wherrett, *The Miracle of the Empty Beds* (Toronto: University of Toronto Press, 1977), 116.

41 P.G. Nixon, "Early Administrative Developments in Fighting Tuberculosis among Canadian Inuit: Bringing State Institutions Back In," *Northern Review*, Winter 1988, 67.

CHAPTER SEVEN

1 R.G. Williamson, interview by A. Grygier, Saskatoon, November 1988.

2 National Archives of Canada (NA), RG85, 78: 201-1(22), "Proposed Itineraries, Season 1947."

3 NA, RG85, 76: 201-1(19); see agreement, 12 July 1944.

4 NA, RG85, 76: 201-1(18), Ross Millar to R.A. Gibson, 4 November 1943.

5 J.W. Anderson, "Peacetime Voyage," *Beaver*, December 1946, 46.

6 NA, RG85, 79: 201-1(25a), memo, J.G. Wright to A. Watson, 22 December 1950; *Arctic* 1, no. 2 (1948): 121; ibid., 2, no. 3 (1949): 200; and ibid., 4, no. 1 (1951): 70–1.

7 NA, RG85, 80: 201-1(26), "Sailing Instructions, CGS *C.D. Howe*," 23 June 1951.

8 Ibid.

9 Ibid., G.E.B. Sinclair to Watson, 27 February 1951.

10 NA, RG85, 78: 201-1(22), memo, Wright to Gibson, 10 January 1947.

11 NA, RG85, 80: 201-1(26), memo, J. Cantley to Wright, 15 December 1951.

12 NA, RG85, 362: 201-1(30), Patrick A. Hill to B.G. Sivertz, 5 October 1954, and R.E. Murdock to Sivertz, 25 October 1954.

13 Ibid., "Eastern Arctic Patrol, 1954, First Part of Voyage," 27 August 1954.

14 Stanley Burke, "Canada's Arctic Ship Dirty and Inefficient," *Vancouver Sun*, 10 September 1954; see NA, RG85, 362: 201-1(30), attachment to letter from J.R. Baldwin to deputy minister, NANR, 18 October 1954.

15 Ibid.

16 Ibid., Sivertz diary, copy in NA&L Branch file, 24 September 1954, with handwritten note on p. 1, "File B.G.S."

17 Williamson interview; confirmed by Sivertz in telephone conversation with the author, September 1990.

18 Betty Marwood, interview with author, Manotick, March 1988.

19 Burke, "Canada's Arctic Ship Dirty."

20 Walter Rudnicki, interview with author, Ottawa, March 1988.

21 R. Banffy, "The Welfare Officer as a Member of the Eastern Arctic Patrol, 1957" (report in Rudnicki files), 2.

22 Based on Williamson, Marwood, and Rudnicki interviews; also author interviews with Titus Allooloo (Ottawa, November 1990), Joanasie Salomonie (Cape Dorset, September 1988), and Alex. Spalding (Toronto, July 1989).

23 Williamson interview.

24 Spalding interview.

25 NA, RG85, 452: 201-1(37), *C.D. Howe* sailing orders, 20 June 1958; and NANR "Instructions to the Officer-in-Charge Eastern Arctic Patrol" and "Guidance Paper for Members of the Eastern Arctic Patrol," in Rudnicki files.

26 NA, RG85, 452: 201-1(37), Dr H.B. Sabean, report on the "Medical Work of the EAP, 1957"; see also letter and interim report (August 1957) Sabean to Dr J.H. Wiebe, INHS, in Rudnicki files.

27 *Northern Affairs Bulletin* 5, no. 3 (April–May 1958): 13–14.

28 Banffy, "Welfare Officer of the EAP."

29 Marwood interview. Marwood also mentioned, however, that the EAP procedures were similar to those of clinics for the poor in the 1950s. As she knew from her previous work experience, "if an indigent person in Hamilton went to those clinics they were all treated like cattle, too."

30 Marwood interview.

31 Dr Brian Brett, interview with author, Ottawa, March 1988.

32 "Arctic Welfare Services," *Canadian Welfare* 38, no. 3 (1962): 111–13 (prepared by the editorial and information staff of NANR).

33 Marwood interview.

34 Williamson interview.

CHAPTER EIGHT

1 Elva Taylor, interview by A. Grygier, Edmonton, November 1988.

2 Jo MacQuarrie, personal communication, April 1989, and Rhoda Innuksuk, personal communication, September 1992.

3 Mini Aodla Freeman, interview by A. Grygier, Edmonton, November 1988.

4 Ibid.

5 Sarah and Simon Saimaiyuk, "Life as a TB Patient in the South," *Inuktitut* no. 71 (1990): 20–4.

6 Titus Allooloo, interview with author, Ottawa, November 1990.

7 *The Camsell Mosaic* (Edmonton: Charles Camsell History Committee, 1985), 94.

8 The medical personnel referred to in this extract are Dr Herbert Meltzer, the medical director and chief surgeon; Drs Matthew Matas,

Margaret Barclay, and William Barclay; and the operating room supervisor, Phyllis Hall.

9 Thoracoplasty is the removal of three or more ribs to collapse a particular area of the lung. In a complete thoracoplasty, as many as eleven ribs might be removed. Pneumothorax is an injection of air into the pleural space in the area of the lung that is most in need of rest. This might be tried before more radical surgery and sometimes was sufficient along with bed rest. Pneumoperitoneum is an injection of air into the abdominal cavity. Crushing the phrenic nerve paralysed the diaphragm, allowing the lung to rest. Resections, or removal of part or all of the lung, were also done.

10 *Camsell Mosaic*, 23–4.

11 Ibid., 248–9.

12 Ibid., 29–30.

13 National Archives of Canada (NA), RG85, 1129: 252-3(3), memo, J.G. Wright to F.J.G. Cunningham, 29 July 1952.

14 Ibid.; see also Cunningham to W.P. Percival, Dept of Education, Quebec, 28 July 1952; and memo, M.L. Manning to J. Cantley, 12 November 1952.

15 See Fred N. Dew, "Report on Education and Rehabilitation in Charles Camsell Indian Hospital," *IHS: Director's Newsletter*, December 1953, 25–30.

16 E. Henderson, "Voice of Santown," *Food for Thought*, April 1949, 21–4, 37.

17 From conversations with A.L. Young, widow of George Young, Kitchener, March–April 1987.

18 NA, RG85, 1474: 252-3(6), R.C. Gagné to J.V. Jacobson, 25 February 1955.

19 Dew, "Report on Education," 27.

20 *Northern Affairs Bulletin* 2, no. 7 (July 1955): 6–7.

21 Frank Croft, "The Changeling Eskimos of the Mountain San," *Maclean's Magazine*, 1 February 1958, 28.

22 *IHS: Director's Newsletter* November 1952, 26–7; and Ruth Cauebaut, "Occupational Therapy in the Charles Camsell Hospital," *Camselletter*, October 1989, 4.

23 "Primary Corner," *The Boar* 22–30 (1955–63).

24 NA, RG85, 1474: 252-3(6), memo, Manning to B.G. Sivertz, 21 May 1954.

25 From answers to the questionnaire survey, 1989–90.

26 Ibid.

27 Dr D. Todosijczuk, interview by A. Grygier, November 1988.

28 *Hamilton Spectator*, 1 December 1952; and NA, RG85, 1129: 252-3(3), H.A. Larsen, RCMP, to director, NA&L branch, DRD, 1 December 1952.

29 Appeeya, for instance, interviewed in Pangnirtung, September 1988, told of a woman who tried to drown herself rather than go out to hospital.

30 Joanasie Salomonie, interview with author, Cape Dorset, September 1988.
31 Ibid.
32 Rev. Brian Burrows interview with author, Hamilton, October 1989.
33 Mini Aodla Freeman, telephone conversation with author.
34 From Todosijczuk interview. See also P.A.C. Nichols, "Enter the European: The Fur Traders," *Beaver*, Winter 1954, 38, for an example of the Inuit superiority to the whites, "who are unable to exist in Eskimo country without a welter of civilized equipment such as heated houses, radios, aircraft, supply ships, and so on, while everything the Eskimo family needs to sustain life in this inexorable country can be carried on a single dog sled."

CHAPTER NINE

1 See, for instance, National Archives of Canada (NA), RG85, 1129: 252-3(1b), letter from "G" Div. RCMP to IHS, 14 October 1949, regarding transportation of a patient from Halifax to Pangnirtung.
2 Brian Brett, interview with author, Ottawa, March 1988.
3 NA, RG85 (Int. 77), 1475: 252-4(1), "Discharge of Eskimo Patients during Winter," extract from E.M. Hinds letter of 8 March 1953.
4 NA, RG85, 1474: 252-3(6), memo, G.W. Rowley to B.G. Sivertz, 28 May 1954.
5 Ibid., R.J. Harries to OC, "G" Div., RCMP, 13 January 1955.
6 Ibid., J.A.H. to Maj. E. Karpetz, 11 March 1955.
7 From Rudnicki files. See also NA, RG85, 1129: 252-3-2, Dr Moore to F.S. Kirkwood, Veterans Affairs, 11 October 1950.
8 Interview with author, Clyde River, September 1988.
9 NA, RG85, 1873: 552-1(2), "Care of Eskimo Convalescent Patients," and NA, RG85 (acc. 2), 463: 1003-1(8), "Relief to Destitute Eskimos," 22 April 1953.
10 NA, RG85 (acc. 2), 463: 1003-1(8), "Interdepartmental Committee on Relief and Tuberculosis Rehabilitation Rations," app. 1, 13 July 1956.
11 See NA, RG85, 1128: 252-3(1a), correspondence between RCMP and IHS, October 1947 to January 1948; and NA, RG85, 1474: 252-3(5), E.H. Copeland to director, NA&L branch, 18 November 1953.
12 Abraham Okpik, interview with author, Iqaluit, September 1988. See also Bishop Marsh's "Cry the Beloved Eskimo" in *Echoes into Tomorrow*, ed. Winifred Marsh (1991), for more examples of the distress caused by carelessness in travel arrangements.
13 Titus Allooloo, interview with author, Ottawa, November 1990. In the early 1960s there was a Children's Receiving Home, or Children's Transient Centre, in the rehabilitation complex at Iqaluit (see NA, RG85, 1934:

252-4/169, J.F. Delaute's memo of 28 April 1961). One wonders if Allooloo would not have been better placed there for his wait to go farther north and why, indeed, he was not so placed.

14 Rev. Brian Burrows, interview with author, Hamilton, October 1989.

15 Ibid. Similar views were expressed by Ralph Ritcey, Ottawa, January 1987. For examples of the administration's attitudes during the late 1940s through the 1950s, see NA, RG85, 78: 201-1(22), A. Stevenson to Gibson, "Report on Relief Expedition S.S. 'North Pioneer' to Eastern Arctic, 1947," p. 3 (sanitation), p. 4 (Eskimo Book of Wisdom), and p. 7 (paragraph beginning "As is well known, this woman ..."). See also the Northern Affairs bulletin North 1, no. 8 (1954): 6; ibid. 3, no. 4 (1956): 13; ibid. 3, no. 5 (1956): 4; ibid. 4, no. 3 (1957): 4; ibid. 5, no. 2 (1958): 10; and ibid. 7, no. 3 (1960): 7. While two of these items urge a nonracist attitude, they reflect a consciousness of the presence of racist attitudes among their readers. That the administrators' attitudes only reflected prevailing community attitudes is suggested by such articles as in Beaver, September 1946, 32–7, 47; Canadian Forum, June 1952, 54–5; Financial Post, 22 June 1957, 25; and Food for Thought, March 1960, 251–3. An excellent and sensitive analysis of the relations between the white administration and the Indians and Inuit, and the consequences of this state of affairs, was given by Dr C.H.S. Jayewardene in his monograph "Crime and Society in Churchill" (Department of Indian Affairs and Northern Development, 1972).

16 Burrows interview.

17 Robert Williamson, interview by A. Grygier, Saskatoon, November 1988; and Alex. Spalding, interview with author, Toronto, July 1989.

18 Williamson interview.

19 Elizabeth, interview with author, Iqaluit, October 1988.

20 From author interviews with Ralph Ritcey, Ottawa, January 1987, and Walter Rudnicki, Ottawa, March 1988. See also, Mary Carpenter-Lyons, "Sarah's Choice," Tribal Reporter, 5 June 1989; and Kirk Lapointe, "TB Threat in North Left Wandering Inuit Tracking their Roots," Globe and Mail, 17 September 1986.

21 NA, RG85, 1129: 252-3(3), Philip Phelan, superintendent of education, Indian Affairs branch, Department of Citizenship and Immigration, to G.E.B. Sinclair, NA&L branch, 19 May 1952. There is a handwritten note by M. Grantham to Mr Cantley on the letter: "Where can this boy be placed? It is apparent he is now a misfit and furthermore the responsibility of this Administration. No doubt he was one of the polio patients from King George Hospital."

22 NA, RG85, 1360: 252-6(1), memo, W. Rudnicki to Sivertz, 27 November 1956.

23 Ibid. See also Rudnicki to Jack Finlay, CAS, 12 June 1958; Rudnicki to Dr Ewart, Mountain Sanatorium, 12 June 1958; Rudnicki to Dr Hayward,

Lady Willingdon Hospital, 12 June 1958; and Finlay to Rudnicki, 6 June 1958.

24 Ibid., attachment to letter from Ewart to Rudnicki, 2 July 1958.

25 Ibid.; see A.H. Stevens to Rudnicki, 8 July 1958; Finlay to Rudnicki, 10 July 1958; and F.W. Thompson to Finlay, 18 July 1958.

26 Betty Marwood, interview with author, Manotick, March 1988.

27 Ibid.

28 See *Ottawa Citizen*, 13 December 1988; *News/North*, 22 May 1990; and *Medical Patient Search Project. Summary: Final Report* (Government of the Northwest Territories, Department of Health, April 1991).

29 Burrows interview. For an example, see NA, RG85, 1129: 252-3(1B), letter from Dr R.N. Simpson, IHS, to the commissioner, RCMP, 6 December 1949, which reads: "Would you kindly have your officer in charge at [Kuujjuaq] advise the relatives of E9 ... that she died on 5 December, 1949, after receiving all possible medical care."

30 See, for instance, NA, RG85, 1129: files 252-3(1B), 252-3(2), 252-3(2A), and 252-3(3), for reports of deaths and burials from April 1949 to December 1952. These include accounts from various funeral and cemetery directors for coffins, plots, and grave digging.

31 Burrows interview.

32 The bulk of these letters are now in the section of DIAND that deals with native claim liaison, constitutional development, and strategic planning.

33 In DIAND collection.

34 See *Medical Patient Search Project: Final Report*.

35 See *Inuktitut* 71 (1990): 30–5; *Edmonton Sunday Journal*, 24 June 1990; and *Hamilton Spectator*, 11 and 13 December 1989.

36 It appears that Orzel could find no records of Inuit patients' burials between that of Mikeyook in December 1952 and March 1955, nor were any Inuit buried at the Roman Catholic cemetery in Hamilton. Presumably, there were no Inuit deaths at Mountain Sanatorium during this period. No departmental records after mid-1953 or hospital records were available to the researcher.

37 Rev. B. Burrows, C. Orzel, and Sheila Meldrum of DIAND, telephone conversations with author, April 1992.

38 Jo MacQuarrie and Cpl. M. Hollett, RCMP, telephone conversations with author, April 1992.

CHAPTER TEN

1 "Health Services Plan, Northwest Territories, 1962–7," in Walter Rudnicki's files.

2 G. Graham-Cumming, "Northern Health Services," *Canadian Medical Association Journal* 100 (15 March 1969): 530. See also H. Brian Brett, "A Synopsis of Northern Medical History," ibid., 523–4.

3 J. Waldo Monteith, "Special Health Problems," *Financial Post*, 10 June 1961, 59; see also Brett, "Synopsis of Northern Medical History," 525.

4 John S. Willis, "Disease and Death in Canada's North," *Medical Services Journal Canada* 19, no. 9 (October 1963): 767.

5 I. Norman Smith, "What's New in the North," *North* 10, no. 3 (May–June 1963): 19–20. See also the decision by the NWT council that it could not afford a plan to lure doctors to the North by guaranteeing a gross income of $30,000 p.a., in *North* 8, no. 1 (January–February 1961): 48.

6 A.M. Bryans, "The Summer School of Frontier Medicine, CAMSI Exchange: Inuvik 1967," *Canadian Medical Association Journal* 100 (15 March 1969): 512–15.

7 S. Grzybowski, K. Styblo, and E. Dorken, "Tuberculosis in Eskimos," *Tubercle* 57, no. 4, supp. (1976): s9.

8 *Annual Report, 1963–64* (Department of National Health and Welfare, Medical Services Branch), 15.

9 L. Black, "Morbidity, Mortality and Medical Care in the Keewatin Area of the Central Arctic: 1967," *Canadian Medical Association Journal* 101 (15 November 1969): 577–81.

10 Grzybowski, Styblo, and Dorken, "Tuberculosis in Eskimos," s8–9.

11 *Report on Health Conditions in the Northwest Territories 1968* (Department of National Health and Welfare, Northern Health Service, 1969), 9.

12 F.H. Hicks, "The Eastern Arctic Medical Patrol," *Canadian Medical Association Journal* 100 (15 March 1969): 537–8.

13 Grzybowski, Styblo, and Dorken, "Tuberculosis in Eskimos," s8.

14 *Report on Health Conditions in the Northwest Territories, 1968*, 8.

15 Grzybowski, Styblo, and Dorken, "Tuberculosis in Eskimos," s28–30.

16 Ibid., s27, for 1960–74. For 1975–83, see *Indian and Inuit of Canada Health Status Indicators, 1974–83* (Department of National Health and Welfare, Medical Services Branch, December 1986), table c13.

17 Grzybowski, Styblo, and Dorken, "Tuberculosis in Eskimos," s34–5.

18 Rudnicki files.

19 Rudnicki, interview with author, Ottawa, March 1988.

20 Ibid.

21 Northern Welfare Service, "Long Term Plans: Review of 1961 Operations and Plans for 1962," 31 January 1962; in Rudnicki files.

22 These, of course, had been started by the missions many years before and had been run by them in conjunction with their hospitals.

23 See correspondence in National Archives of Canada (NA), RG85, 1873: 552-1(2), and NA, RG85, 1475: 252-4-1.

24 This was later raised to $400 per person. But see NA, RG85, 1873: 564-2-1, letter from J.O. Plourde, OMI, to R.A. Gibson, deputy commissioner, NWT, 26 July 1946, asking for a temporary allowance of $500 per person to help cover back debts incurred.

25 See, for instance, NA, RG85, 1475: 252-4-1, memo, J. Cantley to Mr Fraser, 15 July 1953.

26 See correspondence in NA, RG85, 1475: 252-4-3(1) and 252-4-1.

27 NA, RG85, 1475: 252-4-1, memo, Cantley to Fraser, 31 July 1953, sent on to F.J.G. Cunningham, NA&L branch, and H.A. Young, deputy minister, DRD; and exchange of letters between Young and Maj. Gen. E.L.M. Burns, deputy minister, Veterans' Affairs, 5–28 August 1953.

28 NA, RG85, 1475: 252-4(1), Sperry to Dr W. Falconer, 16 November 1953.

29 NA, RG85, 1474: 252-3(5), Moore to Cunningham, 17 December 1953.

30 NA, RG85, 1475: 252-4-1, "Eskimo TB Discharges 1954," from memo, R.A. Vincent to B.G. Sivertz, 12 August 1955.

31 NA, RG85, 1475: 252-4-1, attachment to letter from Moore to Sivertz, 16 December 1955, asking for a meeting to discuss the problem.

32 See NA, RG85, 1279: 252-4/169(1), memos, "Proposed Rehabilitation Center for Frobisher Bay," 24 February 1956, and "Rehabilitation Center, Frobisher Bay," 2 March 1956; and NA, RG85, 1279: 252-4/169(2), memo, "Tentative Policy for the Selection of Eskimo Candidates for the Frobisher Bay Rehabilitation Centre," 5 July 1957. See also *Northern Affairs Bulletin* 4, no. 4 (May–June 1957): 7.

33 NA, RG85, 1279: 252-4/169(2), Cunningham to secretary of Treasury Board, 22 July 1957.

34 Ibid., memos, R.J. Green to R.A.J. Phillips, 20 September and 18 October 1957.

35 NA, RG85 (Int. 95), 1934: A252-4/169, nominal list of residents.

36 Ibid., memo for file, M. Morin, 20 April 1961.

37 Ibid., T. Golding, "Adult Education Classes in Rehabilitation Centre," 13 October 1961.

38 Ibid., memo for file, F.W. Thompson, 27 November 1961.

39 Joy Rutherford, "Rehabilitation: Sofa or Springboard?" *North* 12, no. 5 (September–October 1965): 35–8.

40 Northern Welfare Service, "Review of 1961 Operations," January 1962; in Rudnicki files.

41 R.G. Williamson, interviews by A. Grygier, Edmonton, November 1988, and telephone conversations with author, August 1991.

42 Williamson, telephone conversation with author, August 1991. For more information on this project and its difficulties, see NA, RG85, 1935: A252-4/184, correspondence between Williamson, F.J. Neville, R.L. Kennedy, and C.M. Bolger, April–August 1961.

43 Terry Cook, "Inventory of the Records of the Northern Affairs Program," *Records of the Northern Affairs Program (RG 85)* (Ottawa: Public Archives of Canada, Federal Archives Division, 1982), 17–18.

44 Ibid., 19–22.

45 *Report on Health Conditions in the Northwest Territories* (Health and Welfare Canada, Medical Services, NWT Region, tabled on 16 March 1989), 1–3.

46 Ibid., 1.

47 *Health and Health Services in the Northwest Territories*, a report from the Territorial Hospital Insurance Services Board and the Department of Health (Government of the Northwest Territories, 1990), 29.

48 Ibid., 32.

49 John S. Willis, "Disease and Death in Canada's North," *Medical Services Journal* 19, no. 9 (October 1963): 767.

50 Personal communication, in the Baffin, October 1988. See also Jonathan Cote, "Exiled at Birth," *Alberta Report*, 15 December 1986, 46.

51 Raw data from *Health and Health Services in the Northwest Territories* (Government of the Northwest Territories, 1990), 30. Percentages calculated by the author.

52 Matthew Fisher, "Handicapped Find Friendly Home in Small, Isolated NWT Hospital," *Globe and Mail*, 26 December 1988.

53 *Health and Health Services in the Northwest Territories: Summary* (Government of the Northwest Territories, Department of Health, 1991), 5.

54 "Trends in the Number of New Active and Reactivated Cases of Tuberculosis in Different Population Groups, Canada, 1979–1989" (Health and Welfare Canada, Medical Services Branch, 1991); and *Edmonton Sunday Journal*, 24 June 1990.

CHAPTER ELEVEN

1 See National Archives of Canada (NA), RG85, 1871: 550-1(1A), memo, D.L. McKeand to R.A. Gibson, 25 October 1943.

2 Jean Labbé, *Les Inuits du nord québécois et leur santé* (Quebec: Gouvernement du Québec, Ministère de la Santé et des Services sociaux, 1987), 36.

3 Ibid., 43.

4 No Quebec government figures are available from the Ministère de la Santé et des Services sociaux (MSSS) for 1967, and only the total number of cases is available until 1973. From 1973 on, MSSS provides figures separately for new active and for reactivated cases. No reactivated cases have occurred since 1985. Statistics Canada received notification of (and reported on) only new cases before 1970, new active and reactivated

cases separately 1970–78, and only total (new active plus reactivated) cases from 1979 on.

5 From a telephone conversation with Dr Fernand Turcotte of Projet Nord, Centre hospitalier de l'Université Laval, Quebec, September 1991.

6 Quebec and Newfoundland had early adopted BCG vaccination on a large scale for their general population; it accounted for about 80 and 8 per cent, respectively, of all vaccinations reported in the country for the non-native population in the 1951–61 period. See A.S. Brancker et al., "A Statistical Chronicle of Tuberculosis in Canada: Part I. From the Era of Sanitorium Treatment to the Present"; and *Health Reports 1992* 4, no. 2, Statistics Canada, cat. 82-003, 112.

7 From telephone conversations with Dr André Beauchesne, Santé publique, MSSS, Gouvernement du Québec, September–November 1991.

8 Gordon W. Thomas, "History of Canadian Surgery: Wilfred T. Grenfell, 1865–1942. Founder of the International Grenfell Association," *Canadian Journal of Surgery* 9 (April 1966): 126.

9 W.A. Paddon, "Tuberculosis Control in Northern Labrador" (DPH thesis, School of Hygiene and Tropical Medicine, London, 1957), 10.

10 Ibid., 11.

11 Ibid., 10.

12 Ibid., 12.

13 Ibid., 13.

14 Ibid., 20.

15 Ibid., 23.

16 Gordon Thomas, *From Sled to Satellite* (Toronto: Irwin Publishing, 1987), 43.

17 Ibid., 41, 44. This compares with $7 per day for the mission hospitals in the NWT, but in their case Health and Welfare also paid the doctors' salaries.

18 Paddon, "Tuberculosis Control," 9, 35.

19 Ibid., 31.

20 Although the Moravian Brothers tried to supplant Inuit culture with Christian practices, they helped keep the Inuit language alive by teaching and preaching in Inuktitut. When Newfoundland joined Confederation in 1949, schooling became a government responsibility and instruction in Inuktitut was forbidden. Few young people can now speak it. Only recently has it been reintroduced into the elementary schools, and children in kindergarten through Grade 2 can now enter Inuktitut immersion programs. See Matthew Fisher's article, "Young Natives Losing Link to 'Old Ways,'" *Globe and Mail*, 3 December 1990.

21 Ibid.

22 Bill Bavington, "Tuberculosis Control in Northern Labrador," *Grenfell Clinical Quarterly* 2, no. 2 (1986): 138.

23 Maureen Baikie, "Perspectives on the Health of the Labrador Inuit," *Northern Perspectives* 18, no. 2 (March–April 1990): 21–2.

24 According to census figures from 1961 on, the Inuit make up 0.1 per cent of the population of Canada, yet during 1966–69 they comprised on average 2.9 per cent of the new active cases of TB reported by Statistics Canada. A decade later, Inuit patients made up 0.93 per cent of all new active or reactivated cases. The comparable figures for Newfoundland, where Inuit make up 0.2 per cent of the population, were 3.9 per cent in 1966–69 and 1.25 per cent in 1976–79. See Statistics Canada, *Tuberculosis Statistics: Morbidity and Mortality*, 1966–69, table 10; 1976, table 7; and 1977–79, table 9. (Percentages calculated by the author.)

25 Maureen Baikie, "Tuberculosis in Northern Labrador," *Grenfell Clinical Quarterly* 1, no. 2 (1985): 37–9.

26 From telephone conversations with Dr J.W. Scott, MOH, Grenfell Regional Health Services, September–November 1991.

27 The deplorable conditions in which this unhappy displaced group are living, and the comparison of their present state with that of less than 30 years ago (see *Globe and Mail*, 13 February 1993, D1, D5, and 19 February 1993, A2, A23) underline the importance of emotional well-being and adequate living conditions in combatting tuberculosis.

28 The total number of cases among Inuit in Canada for 1980–84 was 142, in a population of around 23,200 (1981 census). The total number of cases among Inuit in Quebec for 1980–84 was 71, in a population of 4,875 (MSSS, Government of Quebec, 1991). The rate given in table 24 for Labrador Inuit in 1981–85 is a slight overestimate since it was based on a smaller estimate of population than given in the Baikie study.

CHAPTER TWELVE

1 Medical Services Branch, Health and Welfare Canada gives the rates per 100,000 population of new and reactivated tuberculosis cases for 1984–89 as follows: Inuit, 69.9 (average of rates based on minimum and maximum population estimates in 1986 census); native Indians, 74.7 (average of rates based on minimum and maximum population estimates in 1986 census); foreign-born Canadians of Asian origin, 74.8. Since the latter groups, with populations of 500,120 and 692,600, respectively, are much more numerous than the Inuit, they now make up by far the largest groups of tuberculosis patients in Canada: native Indians 17.8 per cent and Asian-born 27.2 per cent in 1987–89. Statistics Canada, however, estimating notification rates by population, shows Inuit as still having the highest rates, followed closely by status Indians and foreign-born Canadians from Asia; see A.S. Brancker et al., "A Sta-

tistical Chronicle of Tuberculosis in Canada: Part II. Risk Today and Control," *Health Reports 1992* 4, no. 3, 283, chart 3.

2 Glenn Tinder, "Can We Be Good without God?" *Atlantic Monthly*, December 1989, 72.

3 See C.H.S. Jayewardene, "Crime and Society in Churchill" (DIAND, 1972), and other references mentioned in chap. 9, n. 15.

4 Gro Harlem Brundtland, *Our Common Future* (New York: Oxford University Press, 1987).

5 See P.G. Nixon, "Early Administrative Developments in Fighting Tuberculosis among Canadian Inuit: Bringing State Institutions Back In," *Northern Review*, Winter 1988.

6 See Terry Copp and Bill McAndrew, *Battle Exhaustion: Soldiers and Psychiatrists in the Canadian Army, 1935–1945* (Montreal: McGill-Queen's University Press, 1990), 42, 58.

7 See Nixon, "Early Administrative Developments," 71, for the difference between Dr K.F. Rogers's 1938 survey report and the official government statement based on it.

8 Maurice Cutler, "Perhaps We Could Have Done Better," *Business Quarterly*, Autumn 1972, 93–4.

A Note on Sources

There were two main primary sources for this book: the archival records of the Northern Affairs Program (National Archives of Canada, RG85) and the interviews with people who took part in the events recounted, either as government workers or officials, or as patients. Both sources were rich in information. The first provided details of the programs, the policies, the "objective" results, and the administrators' views and problems. The second was important for an appreciation of the effects of the programs on the people concerned, the personal impact, and the everyday facts that rarely appear in government documents; and also for alternative views on how the epidemic might have been handled and how the programs were actually implemented.

The questionnaire survey produced some additional material, as did the old Northern Affairs welfare files (now at Indian and Northern Affairs Canada) rescued by Graham Rowley, and the personal files of Walter Rudnicki. The archival records of the Department of Health and Welfare were not searched, but much relevant material originating from that department can also be found in RG85, and additional material was acquired from the Indian and Northern Health Service and Medical Services Branch annual reports in the library of Health and Welfare Canada.

Among the secondary sources tapped, Statistics Canada's annual reports on tuberculosis statistics were, of course, invaluable. The Indian Health Service Director's newsletters and the *Northern Affairs Bulletin* (called *North* from 1960 on) were useful adjuncts to RG85; they also provided some insights into the outlook and attitudes of the government officials of the time.

Books and articles that contributed largely to my knowledge of the background to the events were the following: G.J. Wherrett, *The Miracle of the Empty Beds* (Toronto: University of Toronto Press, 1977); G.W. Rowley, *What are Eskimos?* (Ottawa: Information Canada, 1971); K.J. Crowe, *A History of the Original Peoples of Northern Canada*, rev. ed. (Montreal: Arctic Institute of

North America, McGill-Queen's University Press, 1991); N. and W. Kelly, *The Royal Canadian Mounted Police: A Century of History* (Edmonton: Hurtig Publishers, 1973); J. Labbé, *Les Inuits du nord québécois et leur santé* (Quebec: Gouvernement du Québec, Ministère de la Santé et des Services sociaux, 1987); G. Thomas, *From Sled to Satellite* (Toronto: Irwin Publishing, 1987); and M. Aodla Freeman, *Life among the Qallunaat* (Edmonton: Hurtig Publishers, 1978).

Information more specific to this story was drawn from Diamond Jenness, *Eskimo Administration*, vol. 2, *Canada*, technical paper 14 (Montreal: Arctic Institute of North America, 1964); *The Camsell Mosaic* (Edmonton: Charles Camsell History Committee, 1985); Terry Cook's clear and informative *Records of the Northern Affairs Program (RG 85)* (Ottawa: Public Archives of Canada, Federal Archives Division, 1982); and Dr W.A. Paddon's excellent 1957 account of "Tuberculosis Control in Northern Labrador" (unpublished DPH thesis, London School of Hygiene and Tropical Medicine, U.K.). Dr S. Grzybowski's work on tuberculosis among the Inuit is fundamental to any study of the subject, and I found two of his major studies particularly helpful. The first, with K. Styblo and E. Dorken, was "Tuberculosis in Eskimos," *Tubercle* 57, no. 4, supp. (1976); the second, with A.S. Brancker, D.A. Enarson, E.S. Hershfield, and C.W.L. Jeanes, was "A Statistical Chronicle of Tuberculosis in Canada," a two-part publication by Statistics Canada in cat. 82-003, *Health Reports 1992* 4, "Part I. From the Era of Sanitorium Treatment to the Present" in no. 2, and "Part II. Risk Today and Control" in no. 3.

The Canadian Periodicals Index turned up many interesting articles on the Inuit and on tuberculosis but few directly on the two together. *Arctic, Beaver, Eskimo, Maclean's* and, recently, *Inuktitut* magazines proved most fruitful.

Credits

Material from "Peacetime Voyage," J.W. Anderson, *The Beaver*, December 1946; "Out of the Stone Age," Peter Freuchen, *The Beaver*, September 1951; and "Enter the European – The Fur Trader," P.A.C. Nichols, *The Beaver*, Winter 1954, is published by permission of the publisher.

Material from "The Field Surveys and the Radiographic Department 1946–1966," "Exercise Routines for Tuberculosis Patients," and "Five Years at the Camsell Hospital," which originally appeared in the *Camsell Mosaic*, is published by permission of the Charles Camsell History Committee and the Royal Alexandra Hospitals.

Portions of Kathleen Dier's "Early Days," *The Canadian Nurse/L'infirmière canadienne* 80, no. 1, are reproduced by permission of the publisher.

Remarks by Alma Houston were originally published in "Perhaps We Could Have Done Better," Maurice Cutler, *Business Quarterly* 37, no. 32 (Autumn 1972) and are published by permission of the publisher.

Quotations from "Tuberculosis Control in Northern Labrador," W.A. Paddon, DPH thesis, London School of Hygiene and Tropical Medicine, 1957, are published by permission of W.A. Paddon.

Material from "What Are Eskimos," previously published in *The Arctic Circular* and subsequently in IAND publication no. QS-2013-0000-EE-A-11 by Information Canada, Ottawa, 1971 is published by permission of the author, G.W. Rowley.

Quotations from letters to Louis St Laurent and "Cry the Beloved Eskimo" by Donald B. Marsh (Donald B. Marsh and Winifred Marsh, *Echoes into Tomorrow*, 1991) are published with the permission of Winifred Marsh.

Quotations from "Medical Observations and Problems in the Canadian Arctic," Dr Otto Schaefer, *Canadian Medical Association Journal* 81, 15 August 1959 are reproduced by permission of the publisher.

Material from *The Miracle of the Empty Beds*, G.J. Wherrett (Toronto: University of Toronto Press, 1977) is published by permission of the publisher.

Index